Get ahead!
specialties
OSCEs and Data Interpretation

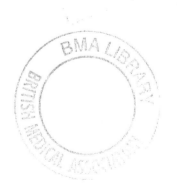

Get ahead!

specialties

OSCEs and Data Interpretation

Nadeem Hasan BM BCh, MA (Cantab), MSc, MFPH, DRCOG
Specialty Registrar in Public Health, London, UK

Caroline Watson BM BCh, MA (Oxon), MRCP
Specialty Registrar in Haematology, Oxford, UK

Joyee Basu BM BCh, MA (Oxon), MRCP
Specialty Registrar in Cardiology, Oxford, UK

Series Editor

Saran Shantikumar BA, BSc, MBChB, MRCS
Academic Clinical Fellow in Public Health
University of Warwick, UK

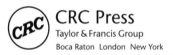

CRC Press
Taylor & Francis Group
Boca Raton London New York

CRC Press is an imprint of the
Taylor & Francis Group, an **informa** business

CRC Press
Taylor & Francis Group
6000 Broken Sound Parkway NW, Suite 300
Boca Raton, FL 33487-2742

© 2016 by Taylor & Francis Group, LLC
CRC Press is an imprint of Taylor & Francis Group, an Informa business

No claim to original U.S. Government works

Printed on acid-free paper
Version Date: 20150603

International Standard Book Number-13: 978-1-4441-7017-7 (Paperback)

Visit the Taylor & Francis Web site at
http://www.taylorandfrancis.com

and the CRC Press Web site at
http://www.crcpress.com

Contents

Acknowledgements

We would like to acknowledge the generous help of the following individuals for their expert content review:

Dr Geetha Anand
Consultant Paediatrician
John Radcliffe Hospital, Oxford

Dr Simon Hampson
Consultant Psychiatrist
Oxford Health NHS Foundation Trust, Oxford

Dr Rakhi Sehmi
GP Registrar, London Deanery
Formerly Specialist Registrar in Obstetrics and Gynaecology
Royal Berkshire Hospital, Reading

Introduction

The Objective Structured Clinical Examination (OSCE) is a core part of the medical curriculum. However, as anyone who has been through them will tell you, doing well in OSCEs can be challenging, requiring a combination of history and clinical examination skills, communication and presentation skills, knowledge of how to interpret clinical signs and form a differential diagnosis and a focused understanding of the further investigation and management of common findings.

Whereas most OSCE revision aids only cover some of these areas, the Get ahead! OSCE guides cover all of them in detail, providing a one-stop shop. As trained OSCE examiners, we also guide you to what the examiners are marking you on, providing sample 'score sheets' for each station, either for reference or to use when practicing.

We take you through the following standard steps in an OSCE:

1. Entering the room and greeting the examiner
2. Greeting the patient and taking the history or performing the clinical examination
3. Thanking the patient and presenting your findings and differential diagnosis to the examiner
4. Answering questions on specific findings, further investigations for your differential diagnosis and management of the condition
5. Thanking the examiner and leaving for the next station

We take you through each history and clinical examination station, step by step, providing example phrases for each question you need to ask the patient. Furthermore, in contrast to the approaches taken elsewhere, we also fully explain why you need to ask each question or perform each examination step, and how to interpret your findings. This will enable you to understand the process of history taking and clinical examination not as a routine to be memorized but as an essential tool in diagnosing the patient, helping you to feel comfortable and in control of each step. At the end of each station, we also provide a 'model answer' for presenting your findings to the examiner to help you with this often challenging part of the station.

Unfortunately for students, most OSCEs do not end with the presentation of your findings. Examiners will follow up with questions ranging from 'Based upon your examination findings, what are the other possible diagnoses?' and 'What would your next steps be in investigating this patient?' to specific questions about the management of the most likely diagnosis. We have included the full range of questions that examiners ask in each station, from the basic areas required for a pass to the more advanced areas and details for students aiming for a distinction. The questions match the syllabus in medical schools throughout the UK, often going beyond this, and are fully in line with current clinical guidelines. Every chapter has been checked by specialists with experience in OSCEs to ensure accuracy and completeness.

Finally, although we are confident that this book will provide you with the knowledge and confidence to pass your OSCEs with flying colours, there is no substitute for experience, so practise, practise, practise!

Nadeem Hasan

1: Obstetrics and Gynaecology

GENERAL GYNAECOLOGICAL HISTORY

Problems in early pregnancy usually come under the topic of gynaecology rather than obstetrics (for example, bleeding and/or abdominal pain in early pregnancy could suggest a miscarriage or ectopic pregnancy). Accordingly, when taking a gynaecological history from a pre-menopausal woman, it is important to always begin by asking: Could this patient be pregnant and could these symptoms be due to problems of early pregnancy?

'Miss C attends the gynaecology outpatient clinic with vaginal bleeding and some abdominal discomfort. Please take a general gynaecological history.'

Score Sheet

Scores: 1 = Not attempted; 2 = Attempted, unsatisfactory; 3 = Attempted, satisfactory

Action	1	2	3
Introduction			
1. Introduces self appropriately, checks patient's name, date of birth and occupation and establishes rapport			
History of presenting complaint			
2. Elicits the presenting complaint and history of presenting complaint and the patient's ideas and concerns regarding her symptoms			
Gynaecological history			
3. Takes a full gynaecological history, including menstrual, obstetric and sexual history			
Past medical history, drug history			
4. Elicits the past medical history, including regular medications and allergies			
Family history			
5. Elicits the family history			
Social history			
6. Elicits the social history			

Continued

Action	1	2	3
Systems review			
7. Completes a systems review			
Summary			
8. Summarizes the findings back to the patient and clarifies any errors, thanks the patient and presents the findings to the examiner			
Overall score		/24	

1. **Introduction.** You should begin all clinical history stations by introducing yourself, checking the patient's details (name and date of birth) and by asking the patient's occupation. This helps to establish rapport and provides information that may be relevant to the underlying diagnosis.

   One approach to taking a gynaecological history is to start by taking down some background details, including:
   a. Whether pregnant or not (always needs to be confirmed with urine pregnancy test [UPT])
   b. Date of last menstrual period (LMP), cycle length, whether regular or irregular and duration of menses (written as, e.g. 4–5/28 regular or 4–5 days every 28 days)
   c. Gravidity and parity (see General Obstetric History section for details)
   d. Use of contraception (hormonal or barrier)

   This allows you to place what follows in context; however, it is equally acceptable to proceed straight to presenting complaint and history of presenting complaint and cover these details then.

2. **Presenting complaint.** This is best done with an open question, e.g. 'What has brought you into hospital today?' List each of the presenting complaints in order and take a focused history for each.

   Common examples include:

Abdominal pain	**Always check whether a woman of reproductive age presenting with abdominal pain is pregnant and do an UPT to confirm. If the test is positive, the diagnosis is ectopic pregnancy until proven otherwise.** Use the 'SOCRATES' tool: **Site:** Where is the pain now/where has it been most recently and is it always in the same place? **Onset:** Is the pain acute or chronic; when did it start; did it come on suddenly, over a minute or so or more gradually; what was the patient doing at the time of onset? When was the LMP and is there any relationship with the menstrual cycle (e.g. dysmenorrhoea during the period, or mittelschmerz mid-cycle) or intercourse (e.g. deep dyspareunia)? Have there been any unwell contacts?

Continued

	Character: What is the nature of the pain (cramping, sharp, dull, burning)? Try not to put words into the patient's mouth, instead document her answer in her own words.
	Radiation: Does the pain radiate anywhere else or is it fixed in one spot? Any shoulder tip pain (suggestive of ruptured ectopic pregnancy)?
	Associated symptoms: Any vaginal bleeding or discharge; any diarrhoea, constipation, nausea, vomiting or change of appetite; any urinary frequency, urgency, nocturia, incontinence, haematuria or dysuria; any dizziness or lightheadedness; or any other associated symptoms?
	Timing: Is the pain constant or intermittent; what is the frequency; is it cyclical (same time every month); are there precipitating factors or is it always there; is it getting better or worse? Any past history of similar pain?
	Exacerbating and relieving factors: Does anything make the pain better or worse; for example, is it better lying still or moving around and is it worse after eating or intercourse? Has she tried using simple analgesia such as paracetamol or co-codamol?
	Severity: On a score of 1–10, how bad is the pain?
Vaginal bleeding	**Always check whether a woman of reproductive age presenting with vaginal bleeding is pregnant and do a pregnancy test to confirm. If the test is positive, the patient will need to have an ultrasound to rule out miscarriage.**
	Onset and timing: When did it first start; what is the relationship to the LMP/menopause/intercourse (is the bleeding intramenstrual, intermenstrual, post-menopausal or post-coital); any possibility of pregnancy; what was the patient doing when it started (intercourse or trauma); how long did she bleed for; has it stopped now; how often is she bleeding; any previous vaginal bleeding?
	Character: Was the bleeding small in volume (spotting) or large in volume; were there any clots; was the patient using pads or tampons or both; how often were the pads or tampons being changed; did the blood soak through onto the patient's clothing?
	Associated symptoms: Any abdominal pain; is it constant or cramping; any vaginal discharge; any dizziness or lightheadedness; any other symptoms?
Vaginal discharge	**Onset and timing:** When did it first start; is it getting better or worse; any history of similar discharge or sexually transmitted infections; any new partners; is the partner experiencing any discharge, itching or other symptoms?
	Character: Colour, volume, consistency, odour, bloodstaining?
	Associated symptoms: Any abdominal pain, vaginal bleeding or itching?

Once you have elicited the patient's presenting complaint(s) and history of presenting complaint(s), it is important to identify her **ideas** and **concerns** regarding her presentation. This will give you additional clues to the underlying diagnosis, will allow you to address the patient's concerns in your further questioning and will allow you to better develop a shared management plan.

3. The full gynaecological history should include (if not already elicited):

   a. **Menstrual history**
- i. Date of first day of LMP
- ii. Menstrual pattern: whether regular or irregular, length of cycle and duration of bleeding
- iii. Amount of bleeding: normal or 'menorrhagia' – bleeding that is unacceptably heavy for the woman, often including clots or 'flooding' or having an impact on daily life
- iv. Use of tampons or pads or both, and duration between changes
- v. Dysmenorrhoea (painful periods)
- vi. Intermenstrual bleeding (IMB, bleeding in between periods) or post-coital bleeding (PCB, bleeding after intercourse)
- vii. Age at menarche (onset of periods) or menopause (if appropriate) and any post-menopausal bleeding (PMB)
- viii. Use of contraception

Causes of abnormal vaginal bleeding		
IMB	**PCB**	**PMB**
Physiological cause: 1%–2% of women spot mid-cycle around ovulation	Vaginal causes: trauma, infection (chlamydia, gonorrhoea, trichomoniasis), malignancy (rare in young women)	**Post-menopausal bleeding should be treated as due to uterine cancer until proven otherwise**
Vaginal causes: infection, malignancy		Vaginal causes: atrophic vaginitis (>90%), trauma, malignancy, infection (chlamydia, gonorrhoea, trichomoniasis)
Cervical causes: infection, malignancy, polyps	Cervical causes: ectropion, infection, malignancy, polyps	
Uterine causes: infection, malignancy, polyps		Cervical causes: infection, malignancy, polyps
Early pregnancy causes: miscarriage, ectopic pregnancy, gestational trophoblastic disease		Other: uterine polyps or carcinoma, ovarian carcinoma, hormone replacement therapy (HRT)
Iatrogenic causes: hormonal contraception, selective serotonin reuptake inhibitors (SSRIs)		

   b. **Cervical smear:** If over 25, date of last cervical smear and result, and any previous abnormal results/colposcopy and outcome

   c. **Obstetric history:** Number of previous pregnancies (gravidity) and those carried beyond 24 weeks (parity), gestation, outcome (live birth, stillbirth, terminations, miscarriages) and mode of delivery

   d. **Sexual history:** Taking a sexual history is a sensitive area, and the depth of questioning should be appropriate to the presenting complaint. At a minimum establish:
- i. If the patient is currently sexually active or has ever been sexually active
- ii. What form of contraception they are using (both partners)

iii. If there is any history of vaginal discharge or itching, superficial dyspareunia (pain at the introitus on initiating penetration) or deep dyspareunia (pain deep in the pelvis on thrusting during intercourse)

If there is any dyspareunia, or if the patient complains of vaginal discharge or itching, then it is necessary to ask further questions:

i. Whether she is with a regular partner or has recently had multiple partners (and if multiple, clarify the contraception used with each)

ii. Whether the patient has previously had any sexually transmitted infections, pelvic inflammatory disease (PID) or has presented with similar symptoms

iii. Whether the partner has/previously had a sexually transmitted infection or any symptoms including discharge, itching, pain or dysuria

Causes of dyspareunia	
Superficial dyspareunia	**Deep dyspareunia**
Vaginal causes: Infection (herpes, chlamydia, gonorrhoea, trichomoniasis, thrush)	PID
	Endometriosis
Vaginal atrophy (post-menopausal) or poor arousal	Adhesions
Lichen sclerosis or psoriasis	Cervicitis
Carcinoma (rare in young women)	
Psychological causes: Fear, ignorance	

Causes of vaginal discharge					
Cause	**Consistency**	**Colour**	**Odour**	**Itching**	**Treatment**
Physiological	Mucoid	Clear–white	Normal	No	Nil
Candidiasis/thrush	Thick/'curd'-like	White	Normal	Yes	Anti-fungals
Trichomoniasis	Frothy	Grey–green	Offensive	Yes	Antibiotics
Gonorrhoea	Watery	Green	Normal	No	Antibiotics
Bacterial vaginosis	Watery	Grey–white	Fishy	No	Antibiotics
Cervical ectropion	Watery	Clear	Normal	No	Cautery/ cryotherapy
Malignancy	Watery	Red–brown	Offensive	No	Dependant
Atrophic vaginitis	Watery	Clear/ blood-stained	Normal	No	Oestrogen

e. **Urinary history:** Any frequency, urgency, nocturia, dysuria or haematuria? Any incontinence/leaking? If so, how severe is it and is it associated with coughing/straining or with urgency? Any dragging sensation down below?

4. The past medical history should begin with any gynaecological conditions, e.g.:

a. Endometriosis: presence of endometrial tissue outside the uterine cavity, which can lead to pain or subfertility

b. Polycystic ovarian syndrome (PCOS): an endocrine disorder leading to polycystic ovaries, anovulatory subfertility and hyperandrogenism

c. Gynaecological malignancies, e.g. endometrial, cervical, ovarian, vaginal or vulval cancers

d. Previous abdominal surgery

e. Urogynaecological conditions (if appropriate), e.g. stress incontinence, urge incontinence or pelvic organ prolapse (the protrusion of the uterus, vagina, bladder, urethra and/or bowel beyond their usual anatomical positions due to weakening of the supporting muscles and ligaments).

The remainder of the past medical history is as for a medical history, paying particular attention to hypertension, diabetes mellitus, stroke, migraine and venous thromboembolism (VTE) (especially with concomitant hormonal treatment, e.g. oral contraceptive pill [OCP] or HRT).

Complete the past medical history with a complete drug history, including prescribed, over-the-counter and 'alternative' medications and details of any allergies and the nature of each allergy. Note any enzyme inducers that may reduce the efficacy of the combined oral contraceptive pill (COCP) for up to 4–8 weeks after stopping. A commonly used mnemonic to remember enzyme inducers is **PC BRAS**:

Phenytoin

Carbamazepine

Barbiturates

Rifampicin

Alcohol (chronic)

Sulphonylureas

Remember also that broad spectrum antibiotics, e.g. amoxicillin, eradicate gut bacteria that normally contribute to enterohepatic cycling of oestrogen and so can cause pill failure.

If the consultation is for early pregnancy, note also any teratogenic medications. Common drugs that are unsafe in pregnancy include:

Non-steroidal anti-inflammatory drugs (NSAIDs)	Closure of ductus arteriosus; fetal oliguria Use paracetamol ± codeine
Warfarin	Teratogenic; fetal haemorrhage Use low-molecular-weight heparin
Tetracyclines	Discolouration of teeth Use safe alternative according to sensitivities
Trimethoprim	Folic acid antagonist Use safe alternative according to sensitivities
ACE inhibitors	Teratogenic; fetal renal failure Use methyldopa
Thiazide diuretics	Fetal thrombocytopaenia Use methyldopa

Continued

Carbimazole	Fetal hypothyroidism
	Low risk, so continue at minimum dose
Propylthiouracil	Fetal hypothyroidism
	Low risk, so continue at minimum dose
Sodium valproate	Teratogenic; valproate syndrome
	Higher risk than others, so consider switching
Carbamazepine	Teratogenic
	Low risk, so balance risk/benefit with mother
Lamotrigine	Teratogenic
	Low risk, so balance risk/benefit with mother
Paroxetine	Teratogenic
	Other SSRIs are safe, e.g. fluoxetine
Lithium	Teratogenic to the fetal heart
	Alternatives difficult; joint care plan needed after discussion with mother

5. Complete a full family history, paying particular attention to gynaecological malignancies that can have a strong inherited component (for example, germline mutations in *BRCA1* and *BRCA2* genes predispose to breast and ovarian cancer, and less commonly to other cancers such as prostate and fallopian tube). Ask also about a family history of hypertension, diabetes, stroke, migraine and VTE, which may be of relevance in contraceptive prescribing.

6. Complete a full social history including a smoking and alcohol history, use of recreational drugs and relationships at home, including any indication of domestic abuse.

7. The systems review should progress through each system in turn as for a medical history, but pay particular attention to each of the common presenting complaints outlined above if not already covered. Complete the systems review by asking if there is anything else that the patient would like to mention, e.g. 'Is there anything that we haven't talked about that you would like to mention or discuss?' This will ensure that you have elicited all of the important facts and will give the patient/actor the opportunity to help you if you have missed anything.

8. Summarize the key findings of the consultation back to the patient to allow her to clarify any errors. Thank the patient and then turn to the examiner to present your findings.

An *example of a presentation* for a patient with primary dysmenorrhoea might be:

Claire is a 14-year-old nulliparous girl who presents with acute lower abdominal pain with the following background: her pregnancy test is negative; her last menstrual period started yesterday, usually regular lasting 3–4 days every 28 days for the last 6 months, with 6 months of less regular cycles before this going back to her first period; she is not sexually active and is not using any hormonal contraception.

She describes the pain as a dull ache coinciding with the start of her period. She has had similar but less severe pains with her last few periods. The pain always settles by the third day of the period and never occurs when she is not menstruating. There is no radiation or associated symptoms, and there are no recent urinary or gastrointestinal (GI) symptoms. The pain eases with ibuprofen but does not go away completely, and she describes the severity as a 7/10.

Onset of menarche was 1 year ago. She has had no intermenstrual bleeding and has never been sexually active and has never had a cervical smear. She is otherwise fit and well with no other gynaecological or medical conditions, has never had surgery, is not on any prescribed or over-the-counter medications other than ibuprofen for the pain and has no allergies. She has no personal or family history of hypertension, diabetes, stroke, migraine or VTE, or any cancers. She has never consumed alcohol, smoked or taken recreational drugs; she lives with her parents and is happy at home and at school.

She is concerned because the pain is really bad this time, and she is worried it is going to keep getting worse; her mum is concerned because she has been sent home from school due to the pain.

In summary, this is a 14-year-old girl, 1 year from the onset of menarche, with suprapubic pain occurring for the first 48–72 hours of her period for the last few periods. These findings are consistent with a diagnosis of primary dysmenorrhoea.

In this case, you may wish to add (for extra points):

The first-line management for primary dysmenorrhoea would be reassurance together with management of the pain with NSAIDs (mefanemic acid or ibuprofen) or, if they are unsuccessful or contraindicated, with the COCP. The Mirena coil intrauterine system (IUS) has also been shown to be beneficial, though it would be a less appropriate first-line treatment in this age group.

CLINICAL SCENARIO: ABDOMINAL/PELVIC PAIN

Acute abdominal pain is normally triaged through A&E to the surgical team, but if the woman is pregnant, the diagnosis is ectopic pregnancy until proven otherwise. If gynaecological pathology is suspected, a gynaecological review will likewise be requested. Chronic abdominal pain of suspected gynaecological origin will usually be referred by the patient's GP directly to gynaecology outpatients.

Diagnosis	Features on history
Acute (early pregnancy related – UPT positive)	
Ectopic pregnancy (see 'Breaking Bad News' scenario)	May be asymptomatic and diagnosed on ultrasound or have any combination of: Lower abdominal pain, which may be central or localized to RIF/LIF, dull or sharp, mild or severe, colicky (initially) or constant (later) Dark vaginal bleeding Rupture may lead to rapid volume loss, shoulder tip pain, hypovolaemic shock and collapse
Miscarriage (see 'Breaking Bad News' scenario)	May be asymptomatic and diagnosed on ultrasound or have any combination of: Lower abdominal cramping 'contraction' pain Vaginal bleeding, which may be heavy or light, with or without passing products of conception (tissue in the blood)
Fibroid degeneration	Increase in size of fibroids during pregnancy compromises the blood supply to the central area of the fibroid causing 'red degeneration' Usually between 12/40 and 22/40 Constant severe pain localized to the site of the fibroid May have low-grade fever
Round ligament pain	Stretching of the round ligaments during pregnancy, occurring in 20%–30% of pregnancies Common in the first and second trimester May be unilateral but more often bilateral on the outer aspect of the uterus Radiates to the groin Exacerbated by movement, relieved by simple analgesia

Remember, of course, that in later pregnancy, abdominal pain may represent (early) labour or Braxton–Hicks contractions.

Diagnosis	Features on history
Acute (not pregnancy related – UPT negative OR positive)	
Ovarian cyst accident	Ovarian cysts tend to be asymptomatic but can cause pain if they twist (tort) or rupture or if there is haemorrhage into a cyst Sudden onset left or right iliac fossa pain Severe haemorrhage may lead to hypovolaemic shock and collapse, requiring resuscitation Torsion of the pedicle may lead to infarction of the ovary/fallopian tube and constant severe pain, requiring urgent surgical detorsion to save the ovary
Pelvic inflammatory disease (PID) (see Case 1 below)	Bilateral lower abdominal pain with deep dyspareunia Abnormal vaginal discharge and/or bleeding History of unprotected sexual intercourse with new/multiple partners History of uterine instrumentation or appendicitis/abdominal infection
Primary dysmenorrhoea	Pain coincides with the start of menstruation, eases after first 24–48 hours of period

Continued

Diagnosis	Features on history
	First presentation common in adolescent girls within 1 year of menarche
	Pain eases with ibuprofen, no pain when not menstruating
Mittelschmerz	Mid-cycle cramping pain due to ovulation
	May be pelvic or clearly localized to one ovary, may change side month to month
	Typically lasts a few hours, though may last up to 48 hours
Non-gynaecological cause	Includes: appendicitis, diverticulitis, strangulated hernia, inflammatory bowel disease, constipation, urinary tract infection and renal stones

Note that exacerbation of any cause of chronic abdominal pain may present as acute abdominal pain.

Chronic

Chronic PID	Persistent infection due to incomplete/lack of treatment of acute PID
	Chronic pelvic pain, vaginal discharge and/or deep dyspareunia
	Subfertility
	Secondary dysmenorrhoea
Endometriosis (see Case 2 below)	May be asymptomatic or have any combination of:
	Pelvic pain, usually cyclical, though may be constant secondary to adhesions
	Dysmenorrhoea, deep dyspareunia, dysuria, dyschezia (pain on passing stool)
	Subfertility
	Rarely cyclical haematuria or rectal bleeding
Adenomyosis	Severe dysmenorrhoea and menorrhagia
	Often with a history of caesarean section or termination of pregnancy (TOP), where the endometrial/myometrial junction has been breached
Adhesions	History of abdominal/pelvic surgery, particularly with multiple procedures
Non-gynaecological cause	Includes irritable bowel syndrome, interstitial cystitis, fibromyalgia, neuropathic pain

Case 1: pelvic inflammatory disease
Presentation

Miss P is a 22-year-old nulliparous woman who presents with acute lower abdominal pain and abnormal vaginal discharge with the following background: her pregnancy test is negative; her last menstrual period was 2 weeks ago, usually regular, lasting 3–4 days every 28 days; she is currently not using any hormonal or barrier contraception.

The pain is a constant dull ache, which started about 3 days ago and has gotten progressively worse; she has never had similar pains before. There is no radiation or associated symptoms, no recent urinary or GI symptoms and, while the pain was eased by paracetamol and ibuprofen at first, they have been less effective over the last 24 hours. The discharge is grey-green in colour but not blood-stained, and has become worse over the last 3 days. She does not have any history of sexually transmitted infections but had unprotected sexual intercourse with a new partner whom she met on holiday in the Caribbean last week but with whom she is no longer in contact.

She has had no intermenstrual or post-coital bleeding, and her periods are not usually heavy or painful. She had been in a monogamous relationship for the last 2 years until it ended last month and, since then, has only had intercourse with the man she met while on holiday last week. She is otherwise fit and well, has not had a cervical smear and has no other gynaecological or medical conditions or history of surgery. She is not on any prescribed or over-the-counter medications other than paracetamol and ibuprofen for the pain and has no allergies. She has no family history of significant disease. She usually drinks 15–20 units of alcohol per week, does not smoke or use recreational drugs and lives in university halls of residence.

She is concerned because she has never had symptoms like this and is worried that she has a sexually transmitted infection.

In summary, this is a 22-year-old nulliparous woman, presenting with a 3-day history of bilateral lower abdominal pain and green–grey vaginal discharge on the background of unprotected intercourse with a new partner last week. These findings are consistent with a diagnosis of pelvic inflammatory disease.

Other possible findings

1. Current: deep dyspareunia, blood-stained discharge, fever.
2. Past medical history: multiple sexual partners; uterine instrumentation, e.g. during gynaecological surgery, childbirth or miscarriage; abdominal infection, e.g. appendicitis.

Questions

1. How would you further investigate this patient?

   Appropriate investigations for suspected PID include: endocervical and high vaginal swabs, bloods including full blood count (FBC) and C-reactive protein and ultrasound if there was suspicion of a tubo-ovarian abscess.

2. What would be the appropriate management in this case?

   The patient should be treated with broad spectrum antibiotics according to local antibiotic guidelines. If the patient is febrile or clinical suspicion of a tubo-ovarian abscess is present, she should be treated as an inpatient with intravenous antibiotics, e.g. a cephalosporin, doxycycline and metronidazole. If the patient is relatively well, she can be managed as an outpatient with oral antibiotics, e.g. ofloxacin and metronidazole (in some centres a stat dose of intramuscular ceftriaxone may also be given).

If there is no improvement after 24–48 hours of antibiotics, the diagnosis should be reviewed, an ultrasound should be performed and a laparoscopy should be considered to investigate for a possible pelvic abscess.

3. What complications of PID are you aware of?

Early complications include formation of a tubo-ovarian abscess and perihepatitis (Fitz-Hugh–Curtis syndrome), which occurs in 10% of patients and presents with right upper quadrant pain due to the formation of adhesions. Late complications include recurrent/chronic PID and chronic pelvic pain, ectopic pregnancy (six times more common after PID) and subfertility.

Case 2: endometriosis

Presentation

Mrs E is a 35-year-old nulliparous woman who has been referred by her GP with chronic severe dysmenorrhoea and deep dyspareunia with the following background: her pregnancy test is negative; last menstrual period was 2 weeks ago, usually regular, lasting 3–4 days every 28 days; and she is currently not using any hormonal or barrier contraception.

The dysmenorrhoea has been present for the last 7 months and starts 3–4 days before her period and continues until the end of the period. The pain is in her lower abdomen and pelvis, and she describes it as much more severe than period pains she used to get, up to 9/10, and lasting much longer. Sometimes paracetamol and ibuprofen ease the pain, but other times they do not, and she has had to take time off work because of it. There is no radiation or associated symptoms and no recent urinary or GI symptoms. The deep dyspareunia is also new, and she describes it as a stabbing sensation on deep penetration, worst just before her period starts. She and her husband have been trying to become pregnant for the last 8 months without success.

She has had no intermenstrual or post-coital bleeding, her periods are not usually heavy and she has had no abnormal vaginal discharge. Her only sexual partner is her husband of 5 years, who is asymptomatic, and she has no past history of sexually transmitted infection or pelvic inflammatory disease. She is otherwise fit and well, and her previous cervical smear last year was normal. She has no other gynaecological or medical conditions or history of surgery. She is not on any prescribed or over-the-counter medications other than paracetamol and ibuprofen for the pain and has no allergies. She has no family history of significant disease. She usually drinks 4–6 units of alcohol per week, does not smoke or use recreational drugs and lives with her husband.

She is concerned because her GP initially advised her that the pain should settle with painkillers, but the pain is so bad that she has had to take time off work most months. She is also concerned that she is unable to get pregnant despite using ovulation sticks to make sure that they are trying at the right time of the month.

In summary, this is a 35-year-old nulliparous woman, presenting with a 7-month history of severe dysmenorrhoea starting 3–4 days before the period and continuing for the entire duration, deep dyspareunia and failing to conceive despite 8 months of trying. These findings are most consistent with a diagnosis of endometriosis.

Other possible findings

1. Current: constant abdominal pain even between periods (due to adhesions); ovulation pain; cyclical or perimenstrual bowel or bladder symptoms, with or without abnormal bleeding; pain on passing stool (dyschezia); and chronic fatigue.
2. Past medical/family history: there is some evidence suggesting an inherited predisposition.

Questions

1. What are some of the common findings on examination in endometriosis?
   In mild disease, examination may be normal but common findings include: pelvic tenderness, a fixed, retroverted uterus (due to adhesions) and enlarged ovaries. Deeply infiltrating nodules are most reliably detected when the examination is performed during menstruation and may visible in the vagina or cervix, or palpated in the pouch of Douglas or on the uterosacral ligaments.

   Patients who experience deep dyspareunia tend to have uterosacral disease, so these would also be tender on examination.

2. What further investigations may be indicated in endometriosis?
   The gold-standard diagnostic test for endometriosis is visual inspection at laparoscopy, unless disease is visible in the vagina or on the cervix, ideally with biopsy for histological diagnosis (though negative histology does not exclude endometriosis). The appearance of endometriosis at laparoscopy is variable and may include: peritoneal lesions presenting as red/black/brown/white 'powder burn' dots; ovarian endometriomas, presenting as 'chocolate cysts' of varying size filled with old blood; and solid rectovaginal nodules.

   Transvaginal ultrasound has a role in detecting ovarian endometriomas, which should be considered for removal to exclude ovarian carcinoma.

   If there is clinical evidence of deeply infiltrating endometriosis, ureteric, bladder and bowel involvement should be assessed, and MRI/ultrasound with or without intravenous pyelogram (IVP) and barium studies should be considered to map the extent of the disease.

   CA125 levels may be raised but have no value as a diagnostic tool.

3. What are this patient's treatment options?
   The first option is empirical treatment of the symptoms without making a definitive diagnosis. Patients who are reluctant to take hormonal therapy, e.g. patients trying to conceive, can often be managed with NSAIDs

and complementary therapies. If this is unsuccessful, or in patients who are happy to take hormonal therapy, ovarian suppression for 6 months can reduce endometriosis-related pain. This can be with progestogens; the COCP, danazol; or gonadotrophin-releasing hormone (GnRH) agonists, though the latter two are associated with more adverse effects and are limited to 6 months' therapy. Symptom recurrence after stopping hormonal therapy is common. The IUS (Mirena coil) also appears to reduce endometriosis-related pain.

The second option is to proceed with laparoscopy and 'see and treat' ablation of endometriotic lesions with laser or bipolar diathermy. This has the added benefit of improving fertility. In cases where the patient's family is complete, as a last resort radical surgery can be considered, with dissection of adhesions, total abdominal hysterectomy and bilateral salpingo-oophorectomy and removal of all visible endometrial tissue. These women will need HRT post-operatively.

4. Where can endometrial tissue be found in endometriosis?
   Endometrial tissue is most commonly found in the pelvis, including the pouch of Douglas, the uterosacral ligaments, ovarian fossae, bladder and peritoneum. Rarely, it can be found in the lungs, muscle and central nervous system.

5. What is adenomyosis and how is it related to endometriosis?
   Adenomyosis is the presence of endometrial tissue within the myometrium and so was previously referred to as 'endometriosis interna'. It can also cause severe dysmenorrhoea together with menorrhagia, and there is normally a history of breaching the endometrial/myometrial junction, e.g. at caesarean section. Diagnosis is by MRI, and treatment is with analgesia and ovarian suppression, though hysterectomy is often required.

CLINICAL SCENARIO: AMENORRHOEA AND OLIGOMENORRHOEA

Amenorrhoea is the absence of menstruation and can be primary (where menstruation has not started by age 16) or secondary (where menstruation has started, and then stops for 6 months or more). Oligomenorrhoea is where menstruation occurs but the cycle is longer than normal (between 35 days and 6 months, at which point it is labelled amenorrhoea). These patients will normally be referred by their GP to outpatient gynaecology. There are several causes, which can be divided between physiological and pathological.

Diagnosis	Features on history
Physiological	
Delayed puberty	Primary amenorrhoea, absence of secondary sex characteristics by age 16, positive family history, diagnosis of exclusion

Continued

Diagnosis	Features on history
Pregnancy	Sexually active (use of contraception does not exclude possibility) Positive UPT
Lactation	Recently delivered and breastfeeding, duration of lactational amenorrhoea varies widely between women
Menopause	Average age in the UK is 52; premature if <45 years old Period of oligomenorrhoea followed by amenorrhoea Hot flushes, night sweats and/or other symptoms of menopause, including headaches, tiredness, change in mood/personality and loss of libido
Drugs (through effect on hormones)	Commonly hormonal drugs, e.g. progestogens, continuous combined oral contraceptives and GnRH analogues. Also antipsychotics can raise prolactin levels, causing amenorrhoea

Pathological

Hypothalamic
(reduced GnRH release leads to reduced FSH/LH, which leads to reduced oestradiol)

Anorexia	See Psychiatry section for full details, but includes: Low body mass index (BMI) with deliberate weight loss and distorted body image Excessive exercise Vomiting after eating, feeling cold, irregular sleeping patterns, poor concentration
Excessive exercise	Excessive exercise without other features of anorexia
Stress	Stress alone can cause hypothalamic hypogonadism
Hypothalamic damage	Through neurosurgery or radiotherapy
Tumour	In adults, more likely to be secondary from another organ; symptoms include: visual field defects, headache, loss of appetite, weight loss, tiredness, euphoric sensations
Kallmann syndrome	Congenital hypogonadotrophic hypogonadism Poorly defined secondary sexual characteristics and anosmia

Anterior pituitary
(reduced FSH/LH release leads to reduced oestradiol)

Pituitary damage	Through neurosurgery or radiotherapy
Tumour	May be a non-functioning macroadenoma (most common), a prolactinoma or a hormone secreting tumour Symptoms depend on hormone secretion and pattern of growth, but local symptoms include: headache, visual field defects, squint, symptoms of hypopituitarism (tends to occur in the following order: LH, GH, TSH, ACTH, FSH), symptoms of anterior pituitary hormonal hypersecretion (acromegaly, hyperprolactinaemia, Cushing disease and thyrotoxicosis)
Sheehan syndrome	Sheehan syndrome is pituitary infarction following postpartum haemorrhage (PPH), therefore look for a history of PPH and symptoms of hypopituitarism

Continued

Diagnosis	Features on history
Ovarian	
Polycystic ovary syndrome (PCOS)	Diagnosis of PCOS requires ≥2 of the following: 1. Oligomenorrhoea or amenorrhoea 2. Hyperandrogenism (clinical and/or biochemical, including hirsutism, acne, alopecia) 3. Morphologically polycystic ovaries on ultrasound (≥12 antral follicles on one ovary or ovarian volume >10 mL)
Premature ovarian failure	Due to premature menopause, as described above
Turner syndrome	45 XO genotype leads to ovarian dysgenesis, short stature and poor secondary sexual characteristics. Other rarer forms of gonadal dysgenesis also exist
Genital outflow tract obstruction	
Congenital causes	Imperforate hymen or transverse vaginal septum present with normal secondary sexual characteristics but primary amenorrhoea due to obstructed menstrual flow leading to accumulation of blood in the uterus (haematometra) or vagina (haematocolpos)
Cervical stenosis	Secondary amenorrhoea with haematometra
Asherman syndrome	Scarring and adhesions, usually following endometrial curettage at evacuation of retained products of conception (ERPC) or termination of pregnancy (TOP)
Female genital mutilation (FGM)	Differs in severity, with the most severe (infibulation) involving the removal of all or part of the inner and outer labia, the clitoris and fusion of the wound leaving a small passage for the passage of urine and menstrual blood
Endocrinopathies	
Various endocrinopathies	Oligomenorrhoea can be secondary to hyperprolactinaemia, Cushing syndrome, hypothyroidism or hyperthyroidism, congenital adrenal hyperplasia or rare virilizing ovarian or adrenal tumours

Case 1: polycystic ovarian syndrome
Presentation

Miss P is a 20-year-old nulliparous woman who presents with irregular periods on a background of a negative pregnancy test and is not currently using any hormonal contraception.

Her last menstrual period was 6 weeks ago, and they have been 2–3 months apart for the last year, lasting 4–5 days. Before this they were more regular and, until she was 17, they were every month. She has been slightly overweight since she was a teenager, but her weight has increased by 3 stone over the last year with most of it in a central distribution. She has also always suffered from acne, which she manages with over-the-counter creams and notes that she developed excess hair on the upper lip, chin and lower back.

She has had no intermenstrual or post-coital bleeding and has not been sexually active for the last year. She is otherwise fit and well, has not had a cervical smear and has no other gynaecological or medical conditions or history of surgery. She is currently using benzoyl peroxide cream for acne but no other medications, and she has no allergies. She has no family history of significant disease. She usually drinks around 25 units of alcohol per week, does not smoke or use recreational drugs and lives in university halls of residence.

She is concerned because she is embarrassed by her weight gain, worsening acne and excess hair and is less able to go out and enjoy herself at university because of it.

In summary, this is a 20-year-old nulliparous woman, presenting with a 1-year history of oligomenorrhoea and obesity, having gained 3 stone this year, associated with worsening acne and hirsutism. These findings are consistent with a diagnosis of PCOS.

Other possible findings

1. Current: amenorrhoea, subfertility, alopecia.
2. Past medical history: family history of PCOS, type 2 diabetes.

Questions

1. What are the Rotterdam criteria for the diagnosis of PCOS?
   The Rotterdam criteria for the diagnosis of PCOS are any two out of the following three:
   a. Oligomenorrhoea and/or anovulation
   b. Clinical and/or biochemical signs of hyperandrogenism (hirsutism, acne, alopecia)
   c. Polycystic ovaries on ultrasound (presence of 12 or more follicles measuring 2–9 mm and/or increased ovarian volume [>10 mL]; not in women taking the COCP)
   And exclusion of other aetiologies (congenital adrenal hyperplasia [CAH], androgen-secreting tumours, Cushing syndrome).

2. What are the long-term complications associated with PCOS?
   The main complications are obesity, insulin resistance and type 2 diabetes, which affects up to 50% of women with PCOS, with 30% developing gestational diabetes.
   In addition to this, extended periods of unopposed oestrogen, as occurs with prolonged amenorrhoea, is a risk factor for endometrial cancer.
   There is currently no evidence of increased mortality with PCOS.

3. What would be the appropriate management of this patient?
   PCOS presents in different women in different ways, and management should be tailored accordingly. Management options can be divided among:
   a. Lifestyle modification: weight loss through diet modification and exercise – this may be enough to ensure resolution of her symptoms.

    b. Managing hyperandrogenism: cosmetic hair removal through shaving/waxing/plucking/creams/electrolysis/laser hair removal; anti-androgens including eflornithine cream, cyproterone acetate and spironolactone; and the COCP (dianette also contains the anti-androgen cyproterone acetate). Metformin also reduces androgen levels through reducing insulin levels.

    c. Regulating periods: COCP and metformin, along with weight loss, can help to regulate periods; 3–4 bleeds per year are sufficient to protect the endometrium.

4. How would you manage this patient if she was trying to conceive?

The initial advice would be weight loss (and smoking cessation if appropriate), which alone may restore ovulation and improve fertility. The first-line drug for ovulation induction in PCOS is clomifene, an oestrogen antagonist, which results in ovulation in around 70% of women and live births in 40%. Clomifene use is limited to 6 months, and cycles need to be monitored by ultrasound to reduce the risk of multiple follicle maturation and multiple pregnancy, which occurs in around 10% of cases.

The second-line treatment options in cases of clomifene failure or resistance include metformin, gonadotrophins and laparoscopic ovarian diathermy:

    a. Metformin is less effective than clomifene but does not lead to multiple follicle maturation, treats hirsutism and increases the effectiveness of clomifene in resistant women.

    b. Gonadotrophins require daily subcutaneous injection and, like clomifene, can result in multiple follicle maturation and so need to be monitored with ultrasound. An additional risk with gonadotrophin-induced ovulation (and rarely with clomifene) is ovarian hyperstimulation syndrome (OHSS).

    c. Laparoscopic ovarian diathermy involves brief monopolar diathermy of a few points on each ovary and is often combined with insufflations of the fallopian tubes with methylene blue to assess patency. It is as effective as gonadotrophin induction of ovulation with lower risks of multiple pregnancy and no risk of OHSS but does require a laparoscopy under general anaesthetic, with its associated risks.

If all the above methods fail, then the patient could be referred for in vitro fertilization (IVF).

CLINICAL SCENARIO: INCONTINENCE

Although not life-threatening, incontinence can have a major impact on a person's quality of life, and urogynaecology is an important field of practice. There are two main causes of incontinence in women: stress incontinence and overactive bladder syndrome, though mixed incontinence, overflow incontinence and fistulae are also uncommon causes. The typical features on history in each include:

Diagnosis	Features on history
Stress incontinence	Leakage of (usually small amounts of) urine with increased intra-abdominal pressure, e.g. coughing, sneezing, carrying heavy loads May have diagnosed/symptoms of prolapse, e.g. 'dragging' sensation Past medical history of any pregnancy, especially if vaginal, prolonged or instrumental, multiparous or post-menopausal
Overactive bladder (OAB)	Urgency ± urge incontinence (usually large amounts), frequency and nocturia ± nocturnal enuresis in the absence of a urinary tract infection May have symptoms of stress incontinence due to bladder contractions with raised intra-abdominal pressure May be precipitated by triggers, e.g. cold weather or sound of running water May be due to bladder neck obstruction after surgery for stress incontinence Rarely secondary to underlying neuropathy, e.g. multiple sclerosis, spina bifida or upper motor neurone lesions
Mixed incontinence	Combination of both symptoms, but diagnosis made after cystometry
Overflow incontinence	Inability to void leads to chronic retention and overflow, with distended bladder/pelvic 'mass' and stress or continuous incontinence May be due to obstruction, e.g. pelvic mass or bladder neck obstruction after surgery for stress incontinence May be due to neuropathy, e.g. diabetes
Urinary fistula	Continuous incontinence Most commonly due to past medical history of obstructed labour/caesarean section by poorly trained personnel in developing countries ('obstetric fistula', though may also be due to sexual violence in populations from conflict zones) Rare in developed countries, secondary to unrecognized complication of pelvic surgery or radiotherapy or malignancy

Case 1: stress incontinence
Presentation

Miss P is a 55-year-old woman who presents with urinary incontinence with the following background: she is G2P2, both children delivered vaginally at term with no complications more than 20 years ago; she is post-menopausal with her last menstrual period 5 years ago; she is not taking any HRT.

She first noticed the symptoms 6 months ago with small volumes of urine being lost when she sneezed during hay fever season and has since noticed it happening with coughing and, more recently, when picking up heavy bags of shopping. She has no symptoms of urgency, frequency, nocturia or nocturnal enuresis, has not noticed any dragging sensation and has not had a urinary tract infection in the last year.

She is otherwise fit and well, her last cervical smear this year was normal and she has no other gynaecological or medical conditions or history of surgery. She is currently not using any other medications and has hay fever but no other allergies. She has no family history of *significant disease. She usually drinks around 10 units of alcohol a week, does not smoke or use recreational drugs and lives at home with her husband. She drinks about six glasses of water or juice per day, and she has a cup of tea in the morning and coffee in the afternoon.*

She is concerned because she thought it would just go away, but it is actually getting worse to the point that she is now wearing pads, and she is embarrassed by the smell.

In summary, this is a 55-year-old post-menopausal woman, presenting with a 6-month history of small volumes of urinary incontinence with sneezing, coughing and lifting heavy bags, on a background of two previous vaginal deliveries at term. These findings are consistent with a diagnosis of stress incontinence.

Other possible findings

1. Current: 'dragging sensation' of uterine prolapse.
2. Past medical history: instrumental or obstructed labour.

Questions

1. What is the mechanism of incontinence in stress incontinence?

   Stress incontinence occurs when increased intra-abdominal pressure (IAP) leads to the intravesical pressure exceeding the closing pressure of the urethra. If the bladder neck is above the pelvic floor, as is normally the case, then both bladder and bladder neck are equally compressed by raised IAP, preventing outflow of urine. However, if the pelvic floor is weakened, then the bladder neck slips through and is no longer compressed when IAP rises. Therefore, the increased IAP compresses the bladder, increasing intravesical pressure, which then exceeds the urethral pressure with resultant incontinence.

2. What investigations might be indicated in this patient?

   A urine dip should be performed and, if positive, a mid-stream urine sample should be sent for microscopy, culture and sensitivity to rule out urinary tract infection. A bladder diary should be provided to the patient for at least 3 days to get a better idea of the pattern of voiding.

   The only way to confirm the diagnosis is to perform urodynamic studies, but this is usually reserved for cases of stress incontinence for patients being considered for surgery to check for any coexisting detrusor instability (see scenario below for description of urodynamic studies).

3. What are the management options available for this patient?

   There are three broad management options: conservative, medical and surgical.

   Conservative management should start with advice to lose weight, quit smoking (chronic cough), manage constipation (straining) and avoid excessive fluid intake and caffeinated drinks as appropriate. The mainstay of conservative management is pelvic floor muscle training (PFMT) of at least eight contractions, three times per day for at least 3 months under the guidance of a trained physiotherapist. If this is beneficial, it should be followed up with an exercise programme. Vaginal 'cones' or sponges of increasing weights are often used to increase muscle strength and are effective in more than 50% of patients.

If conservative management fails, the recommended second-line treatment is surgery. However, medical management with duloxetine may be more appropriate if surgery is contraindicated or if the patient prefers trying medical management first. Duloxetine is a serotonin–norepinephrine reuptake inhibitor (SNRI). Its use is often limited by side effects including nausea, GI upset and headache, and the patient needs to be warned about this.

Surgery should only be performed after urodynamic studies have excluded an OAB because any detrusor overactivity may be made worse. The first-line procedure, according to current National Institute for Health and Care Excellence (NICE) guidelines (published 2006), is a retropubic mid-urethral tape procedure with polypropylene mesh, such as the tension-free vaginal tape (TVT) or trans-obturator tape (TOT). These are effective in more than 90% of cases and can be carried out under general, regional or local anaesthesia. Second-line options include the open Burch colposuspension and autologous rectus fascial sling, both of which are associated with increased morbidity, resources and recovery times compared with TVT/TOT.

In elderly patients or those who wish to avoid surgery, a further option is injection with intramural bulking agents, including glutaraldehyde cross-linked collagen and silicone. These have a lower efficacy than surgery that diminishes with time; repeat injections may be necessary but are associated with low morbidity.

4. What are the main complications associated with the TVT procedure?
   The major risk of the TVT procedure is a 5%–10% risk of bladder injuries, and this is much lower with the TOT approach. Cystourethroscopy is carried out during the TVT procedure to check for bladder perforation, though studies show that bladder perforation does not have long-term sequelae if managed appropriately.

   Further risks include bladder neck obstruction due to the tape being too tight, worsening of OAB symptoms, erosion of the mesh into the urethra and vagina, and bleeding and infection (including urinary tract infection, which occurs in up to 20% of patients within 6 weeks of the procedure).

5. What are the indications for urgent referral in urinary incontinence in women?
   Urgent referral should be arranged if there is any of the following:
   a. Microscopic haematuria and aged over 50
   b. Macroscopic haematuria
   c. Recurrent/persisting urinary tract infection with haematuria and aged over 40
   d. Suspected urinary tract malignancy

Case 2: overactive bladder

Presentation

> *Miss O is a 70-year-old woman who presents with urinary incontinence with the following background: she is nulliparous, postmenopausal with her last menstrual period 20 years ago, and she is not taking any HRT.*
>
> *She first noticed the symptoms 4 months ago with symptoms of urgency and urge incontinence. She has since also noticed increased frequency and has had a few episodes of nocturnal enuresis, though this has been less of a problem since she cut down her fluid intake in the evening. She has not experienced any urinary loss with coughing or straining and has not had a urinary tract infection in the last year.*
>
> *She is otherwise fit and well and has no other gynaecological or medical conditions or history of surgery. She is currently not using any other medications and has no allergies. She has no family history of significant disease. She does not drink alcohol or smoke and lives at home with her sister. She drinks about five to six glasses of water or juice per day, and she has two to three cups of tea every day.*
>
> *She is concerned because she is embarrassed by her symptoms and has been reluctant to leave the house to socialize with friends for fear of not being able to make it to the toilet in time.*
>
> *In summary, this is a 70-year-old woman, otherwise fit and well, presenting with a 4-month history of urinary urgency and urge incontinence with episodes of nocturnal enuresis and no symptoms of stress incontinence or urinary tract infection. These findings are consistent with a diagnosis of overactive bladder.*

Other possible findings

1. Current: symptoms of stress incontinence due to bladder contractions provoked by increased IAP, triggers, e.g. cold weather or running water.
2. Past medical history: surgery for stress incontinence, underlying neuropathy, e.g. multiple sclerosis.

Questions

1. What is the relationship between 'overactive bladder' and 'detrusor overactivity'?

   Overactive bladder is a clinical diagnosis and is defined as urgency with or without urinary incontinence, usually with frequency and nocturia. Detrusor overactivity is a urodynamic diagnosis and is characterized by involuntary detrusor contractions during the filling phase of cystometry, which may be spontaneous or provoked. The symptoms of overactive bladder are suggestive of detrusor overactivity but can also have other causes – not all women with overactive bladder will have detrusor overactivity and vice versa.

2. What investigations might be performed in this patient?

A urine dip should be performed and, if positive, a mid-stream urine sample should be sent for microscopy, culture and sensitivity to rule out urinary tract infection. A bladder diary should be provided to the patient for at least 3 days to get a better idea of the pattern of voiding.

Urodynamic assessment with cystometry is necessary to make the diagnosis but is usually reserved until after a trial of conservative management. Cystometry involves placing a catheter in the bladder to fill and measure bladder (intravesical) pressure, placing a pressure transducer in the rectum or vagina to measure IAP and calculating the detrusor pressure as: bladder pressure – IAP. These pressures and urine flow are recorded with retrograde bladder filling and with a forced cough.

  a. In normal patients, there is no change in detrusor pressure and no urine flow with either filling or coughing.

  b. In patients with detrusor overactivity, there will be no change in detrusor pressure with coughing. However, during filling there will be a spontaneous spike in bladder pressure (i.e. involuntary detrusor contraction), leading to the sensation of urgency and then incontinence.

  c. In patients with stress incontinence, there will be no change in detrusor pressure with either filling or coughing. However, during coughing there will be small-volume urinary flow in the absence of detrusor contraction.

There is no change in detrusor pressure with coughing because both bladder pressure and IAP rise equally and detrusor pressure = bladder pressure – IAP.

3. What are the management options in overactive bladder syndrome?

The management options are: conservative, medical and surgery.

Conservative management should start with advice to lose weight and avoid excessive fluid intake and caffeinated drinks as appropriate. The mainstay of conservative management in OAB is bladder training for at least 6 weeks, increasing intervals between voiding.

Medical management involves using anticholinergics or topical oestrogens. The first-line treatment is oxybutynin and, if not tolerated, alternatives include tolterodine, solifenacin or other anticholinergics. Side effects include dry mouth, constipation, blurred vision and dizziness and palpitations. In post-menopausal women with vaginal atrophy, topical oestrogens can relieve symptoms.

If this is ineffective, the options include: cystoscopic injection of botulinum A toxin into the bladder every 6–12 months to treat idiopathic detrusor overactivity, though long-term data are lacking and the patient has to be willing and able to self-catheterize because there is a risk of total bladder paralysis; sacral nerve stimulation; augmentation cystoplasty; and finally, urinary diversion if all other options have failed or are inappropriate/unacceptable.

DISCUSS CONTRACEPTION OPTIONS WITH A PATIENT

'You are an FY1 in general practice. Miss C is a 19-year-old patient who has made an appointment to discuss her contraception needs. Counsel her regarding her options.'

Score Sheet

Scores: 1 = Not attempted; 2 = Attempted, unsatisfactory; 3 = Attempted, satisfactory

Action	1	2	3
1. Introduces self, checks patient's name, date of birth and occupation and establishes rapport			
2. Clarifies reason for consultation and elicits ideas, concerns and expectations			
3. Takes brief targeted history relevant to prescribing contraception			
4. Explains advantages and disadvantages of different contraception options			
5. Addresses concerns and questions appropriately			
6. Provides written leaflet and checks understanding			
7. Summarizes and closes appropriately			
Overall score		/21	

1. Begin every consultation by introducing yourself and checking that you are speaking to the right patient by asking patient's name and date of birth. Checking the patient's occupation provides additional information that may be useful and also helps to build rapport.

2. Clarifying the reason for the consultation is important to set the context for the following discussion and to build rapport. Start with an open question, e.g. 'How can I help today?'

   It is then important to establish the patient's **ideas** about contraception: Is she currently using any forms of contraception or has she done so in the past and does she have an idea of the type of contraception she wants to use? Is the reason that she is requesting contraception because she or her partner has a sexually transmitted infection (STI; only barrier contraception will protect against STIs)?

   > *Are you currently sexually active? And are you using any form of contraception at the moment or have you ever done so in the past? And do you have an idea of what sort of contraception you would like to use? And have you and your partner been screened for sexually transmitted infections?*

   Move on to asking the patient about any particular **concerns** she may have regarding the discussion and then establish her **expectations** for the consultation, which should include:

   a. Checking whether there are any contraindications to hormonal contraception

b. Explaining the different types of contraception available and their advantages and disadvantages

c. Agreeing on a suitable contraceptive to prescribe

3. Before prescribing the COCP or the progesterone only pill (POP), the Faculty of Sexual and Reproductive Health (FSRH) guidelines recommend that you should check:

a. Blood pressure, BMI and current and past medical conditions, drugs and family history

b. Specifically, whether the patient has ever suffered from any cancer, liver disease, gestational trophoblastic neoplasia, migraine and cardiovascular risk factors (smoking, obesity, hypertension, thrombophilia, previous VTE and hyperlipidaemia)

    i. The use of COCP is an 'unacceptable health risk' if: personal history of VTE/thrombophilia, BP ≥160/95, migraine with aura, current breast cancer

    ii. The use of COCP is 'not recommended' if: ≥35 years and a smoker, BP ≥140/90, BMI ≥35 kg/m² or liver disease

    iii. The use of POP is an 'unacceptable health risk' if: current breast cancer

    iv. The use of POP is 'not recommended' if: previous breast cancer, gestational trophoblastic neoplasia or liver disease

The FSRH additionally advises that prior to prescribing an intrauterine contraceptive (intrauterine copper device [IUCD] or Mirena IUS), a sexual history should be taken to ascertain whether the patient is at higher risk of STIs (<25 years or >25 years and new sexual partner, >1 partner last year, regular partner has other partners) so that they can have swabs taken prior to insertion.

4. The advantages and disadvantages of each of the common methods of contraception are summarized in this table:

Type	Advantages	Disadvantages
Combined oral contraceptive (COC, COCP)	Very effective (0.2–0.3 failures per 100 woman-years) May reduce menstrual blood loss and dysmenorrhoea Reduced risk of ovarian and endometrial cancer (continues several decades after stopping) and colorectal cancer May improve acne May reduce menopausal symptoms	Approximately doubles risk of VTE (though absolute risk remains very low) Small increased risk of ischaemic stroke Small increased risk of breast and cervical cancer Side effects include irregular bleeding, headaches and mood changes
Progesterone only pill (POP)	Can be used in most situations where COCP is contraindicated and no increased risk of thrombosis	Must be taken at the same time every day Less effective than COCP (higher failure rate)

Continued

Type	Advantages	Disadvantages
	Fewer side effects as no oestrogen	Side effects include irregular bleeding and mood changes
Injectable progestogen (Depo-Provera)	Very effective (<1 failure per 100 woman-years) and lasts 12 weeks	Side effects include irregular bleeding, prolonged amenorrhoea and subfertility after stopping and decreased bone density during use
Progestogen implant (Implanon)	Very effective (<0.1 failure per 100 woman-years) and lasts 3 years	Side effects include irregular bleeding
Intrauterine copper device (IUCD)	Very effective (0.6–0.8 failures per 100 woman-years) Can also be used as emergency contraception	May increase menstrual bleeding or dysmenorrhoea or cause irregular bleeding Increased risk of pelvic infection in those with asymptomatic STIs and ectopic pregnancy May cause perforation at time of insertion or be expelled following insertion
Intrauterine levonorgestrel-releasing system (IUS or Mirena coil)	Very effective (0.18 failures per 100 woman-years) and lasts 5 years Decreases menstrual loss and dysmenorrhoea	Irregular bleeding May be expelled
Barrier methods, e.g. male condom, female condom, diaphragm and cervical cap	Condoms offer protection against STIs including HIV, particularly the male condom Diaphragms and cervical caps offer some protection against PID Can be used at the same time as hormonal contraception	Less effective than hormonal methods and user dependant

5. Common questions when discussing contraception include:

   Q: When do I start taking the COCP?

   A: The COCP can be started up to day 5 of the cycle without the need for additional contraception. If the patient is sure that she is not pregnant (or a UPT on the day is negative), then the COCP can be started any time after day 5, but other contraception (e.g. barrier methods) should be used during intercourse for the next 7 days.

   Q: What happens if I miss a pill?

   A: With the COCP, if you miss one pill, you should take a pill as soon as possible (even if it means taking two pills in 1 day) and then continue taking the rest of the pack as usual; you will not need any additional protection.

If two or more pills are missed, then take the last pill missed as soon as possible (leave any earlier missed pills), continue with the rest of the pack as normal and use other contraception (e.g. barrier methods) during intercourse for the next 7 days. If the missed pills are in week 1 of the pack, you will also need to consider emergency contraception if you have had unprotected sex. If seven or more pills are left in the pack (days 1–14), then complete the pack and have the 7-day break as normal. If less than seven pills are left in the pack (days 15–21), then omit the pill-free interval and go straight into the next pack.

With the POP, if the pill is missed by more than 3 hours (12 hours for cerazette), then another pill should be taken as soon as possible and other contraception (e.g. barrier methods) should be used for 48 hours.

Q: If I'm taking antibiotics at the moment, will the pill still work?

A: It used to be the case that patients on the COCP were advised that, if taking antibiotics, they needed to use other methods of contraception (e.g. barrier methods). Since 2011, this advice has been updated in line with clinical evidence, and now no extra contraception is recommended. The advice with the POP has always been that there is no change in efficacy with antibiotics.

However, if you are taking any drugs that come under the class of 'enzyme inducers' (remember PC BRAS, see General Gynaecological History), then you should ideally switch to injectable/intrauterine progesterone.

Additionally, if you have a vomiting or diarrhoeal illness, then you should continue to take the pill but use additional contraception (e.g. barrier methods) for 7 days after the illness has ended.

Always provide a written leaflet with most of the information covered during the consultation that the patient can look at once she gets home. Check that the patient has understood the discussion, and offer her a chance to ask any further questions.

6. Summarize the discussion before thanking the patient and providing details of where to seek help if there are any problems, which in this case would be from the information leaflet, her local pharmacist or her GP.

DISCUSS THE MANAGEMENT OF MENORRHAGIA

'Miss G, a 20-year-old woman, has come to see you in clinic to discuss management options for her heavy periods. You have established that her periods are interfering with her daily life, she is otherwise fit and well, an ultrasound has ruled out local causes and she is not anaemic. Her concern is that her heavy periods are interfering with her work, and she would like to bring them under control. Talk me through your approach to managing her symptoms.'

Score Sheet

Scores: 1 = Not attempted; 2 = Attempted, unsatisfactory; 3 = Attempted, satisfactory

Action	1	2	3
1. Establishes the woman's contraceptive needs and current contraception			
2. Discusses treatment options for a patient who is trying to conceive			
3. Discusses treatment options for a patient who is not trying to conceive			
4. Discusses surgical options in the absence of fibroids			
5. Discusses surgical options in the event that the ultrasound had shown fibroids			
6. Shows an appreciation for the importance of reaching a shared management plan			
Overall score		/18	

1. The key preliminary question in discussing the management of menorrhagia is whether the patient is trying to conceive. If the answer is yes, then clearly contraceptive options are not appropriate. However, if the answer is no, contraceptive options not only provide the double benefits of reducing menstrual flow and acting as a contraceptive but are also more effective.

2. The only non-surgical treatments available for a patient who is trying to conceive are mefanemic acid and tranexamic acid.

   a. **Mefanemic acid** is a non-steroidal anti-inflammatory drug (NSAID) that reduces menstrual loss (by about 30%) through inhibition of prostaglandin synthesis, and is also an analgesic effective for dysmenorrhoea (painful periods).

   b. **Tranexamic acid** is an antifibrinolytic that reduces menstrual loss (by about 50%) through inhibition of fibrinolysis.

   Both drugs tend to be initiated with the start of menses and used only for the duration of the period.

3. The first-line treatment for a patient who is not trying to conceive and who does not plan to try to for more than a year is the **progesterone-impregnated intrauterine system (IUS)**. This is a T-shaped plastic frame, containing the progestogen levonorgestrel, which sits in the uterus. This reduces menstrual loss (by >90%) through the local effect of the progestogen on the endometrial lining. Insertion is by a trained doctor or nurse; the woman can expect irregular bleeding for the first 6 months and, after 12 months, most women will only have a light bleed for 1 day per month, with 20% of women having no bleeding at all. It lasts 5 years without having to be replaced and is a very effective contraceptive with <1/100 women with the IUS in situ becoming pregnant per year. Women can become pregnant as soon as it is removed, so it is a suitable treatment for young women who do not want to start a family, as well as for older

women who have completed their family. Contraindications to the IUS include: breast cancer within the previous 5 years, very large fibroids and untreated pelvic infection.

Note that it is important to distinguish the IUS, synonymous in the UK with the Mirena coil, from the **copper intrauterine contraceptive device (IUCD)**, which can increase menstrual loss.

If the IUS is contraindicated, or if the patient would like to explore other options for personal reasons, then the second-line treatments are mefanemic acid and tranexemic acid as described above. Another option for women who are not trying to conceive is the COCP, though (1) the data on their efficacy in reducing menstrual loss is poor and (2) their use is limited by contraindications and side effects, particularly in older patients.

Third-line therapies include:

a. **Oral or parenteral progesterone (norethisterone)**, normally from days 5–26 in a 27-day cycle, with withdrawal bleeds that are less heavy than the periods occurring on the off days.

b. **GnRH agonists**, with 'add-back' hormone replacement therapy (HRT) if used for >6 months. GnRH agonists will also be accompanied by withdrawal bleeds.

4. Fibroids, also known as leiomyomata, are benign tumours of the smooth muscle layer of the uterus (myometrium). They are common, affecting at least 25% of women, but they vary in size from millimetres to huge fibroids that fill the whole abdominal cavity and so vary from being completely asymptomatic to causing dysmenorrhoea, menorrhagia and local mass effects, e.g. urinary retention and subfertility. They are oestrogen dependent and so regress after the menopause.

In the **absence** of fibroids, there are two surgical options:

a. **Endometrial ablation:** This is the first-line treatment if the uterus is <10 weeks' gestation to palpate. It involves removal or destruction of endometrial tissue together with the superficial myometrium, preventing future endometrial growth and reducing fertility but not sterilizing the patient. There are various methods, including transcervical resection of the endometrium (TCRE) with a monopolar diathermy cutting loop, transcervical rollerball ablation, microwave endometrial ablation and balloon thermal endometrial ablation. It is important that the patient continues to use contraception after ablation and, if the patient consents, an IUS is often inserted at the time of the ablation.

b. **Hysterectomy:** This is clearly the last resort because it will result in irreversible sterilization of the patient. It should be reserved for those cases where all other treatments have been tried and failed and where the woman has completed her family. An ovarian-conserving approach should be employed unless otherwise indicated.

5. In the **presence** of fibroids, there are four surgical options:
   a. **Myomectomy:** This is the removal of fibroids from the myometrium. The approach can be laparoscopic or open depending on the location and size of the fibroids and the experience of the surgeon.
   b. **Transcervical resection of fibroid (TCRF):** Similar to the TCRE but limited to removing the fibroid(s), usually limited to fibroids <3 cm in diameter. This can be extended to TCRE if fertility is not an issue.
   c. **Uterine artery embolization (UAE):** This is the use of interventional radiology to embolize the arteries feeding the fibroid via a femoral approach, leading to shrinking of the fibroid over the following 6–9 months. There is a theoretical risk of placental insufficiency with a pregnancy following UAE, but otherwise the evidence shows that it is a good alternative to a hysterectomy.
   d. **Hysterectomy:** Again, only as a last resort.
6. It is important to counsel the patient as to all the available options and reach a shared management plan together. With regard to the medical options, it is imperative to take into account the patient's needs regarding contraception and childbirth, and it is likewise important to take into account that some women may be uncomfortable with the idea of an IUS and second-line agents may be more appropriate. Likewise, with regard to surgical options, the effect on fertility must be discussed fully before any decision is made; it is likely that the patient will need time at home to consider the implications before coming to a final decision.

Always close by summarizing and checking that the patient has understood the content of the consultation, and thank the patient, making arrangements for a follow-up at the appropriate time. Demonstrating an awareness of these aspects of the consultation to the examiner will help you achieve higher marks in the exam.

DISCUSS THE PROS AND CONS OF HORMONE REPLACEMENT THERAPY

'Mrs P, a 50-year-old woman, has been experiencing hot flushes and night sweats on a background of 3 months of irregular periods. She has been advised by her GP that she may benefit from HRT and has come in to discuss this further with you.'

Score Sheet

Scores: 1 = Not attempted; 2 = Attempted, unsatisfactory; 3 = Attempted, satisfactory

Action	1	2	3
1. Introduces self, checks patient's name, date of birth and occupation and develops rapport			
2. Clarifies history of presenting complaint			
3. Elicits patient's pre-existing ideas, concerns and expectations regarding HRT			

Continued

Action	1	2	3
4. Explains HRT to patient together with pros and cons using simple language			
5. Answers common questions regarding HRT appropriately			
6. Provides leaflets with further information and support groups			
7. Summarizes and closes consultation appropriately			
Overall score		/21	

1. Start any consultation with a patient by introducing yourself and making sure that you are seeing the correct patient by checking patient's name and date of birth. Checking patient's occupation gives you additional information and also helps to build rapport.
2. In a discussion station, the focus is on your communication skills rather than on history taking. However, clarifying the history of the presenting complaint is important to set the context for the following discussion and to build rapport. Start with an open question, e.g.:

> *I understand that you've been to see your GP with some symptoms that have been troubling you; could you tell me a little bit more about these? ... And what did your GP advise you regarding these symptoms?*

In order to appropriately counsel a patient regarding menopausal and perimenopausal symptoms and HRT, it is important to establish some key aspects of the history:
   a. Menstrual symptoms: date of last menstrual period, regular or irregular periods, onset and timing of irregular periods?
   b. Vasomotor symptoms: any hot flushes, night sweats, or sleep disturbance?
   c. Urogenital symptoms: any vaginal dryness, or dyspareunia? Any frequency, urgency, nocturia or incontinence?
   d. Sexual symptoms: any change in libido or sexual function?
   e. Has the patient had a hysterectomy or does she still have her uterus?
   f. Past medical history, including history of breast/endometrial cancer.
   Vasomotor symptoms indicate the need for systemic therapy, urogenital symptoms indicate the need for topical therapy and sexual symptoms may indicate that androgenic therapy may be beneficial. Whether the patient has a uterus will determine the HRT regime that is appropriate.
3. In order to pitch the discussion appropriately and address the patient's specific concerns in your explanation, you should begin by establishing the patient's pre-existing ideas, concerns and expectations regarding HRT, e.g.:

> *You mentioned that your GP discussed that you may benefit from hormone replacement therapy or 'HRT' – can you tell me what you understand by that? And do you have any specific concerns or worries regarding HRT? And can I ask what your expectations are from HRT?*

4. When explaining medical diagnoses and treatments, use simple, jargon-free language and pace yourself appropriately, responding to verbal and non-verbal cues from the patient. Your explanation of HRT should be adapted to the patient's prior understanding and symptoms but as a template:

> Hormone replacement therapy, or HRT, is the replacement of the hormones that are naturally produced by your ovaries until the menopause and then cease after that time. There are two hormones that your ovaries produce: oestrogen and progesterone.
>
> The symptoms of the menopause are caused by a fall in the level of oestrogen in your body. In women who have had a hysterectomy and who no longer have a uterus, only the oestrogen needs to be replaced in order to manage the symptoms. In women who still have their uterus, the progesterone also needs to be replaced. This is because there is an increased risk of uterine cancer if oestrogen is given without progesterone.
>
> For symptoms that affect the whole body, such as hot flushes and night sweats, the hormone replacement can be via tablets, patches or implants under the skin. If you are only experiencing symptoms such as dryness, pain during sex or urinary problems, then hormone replacement is via a vaginal cream, gel, tablet or ring.

A template for explaining the benefits of HRT is:

> There are four major benefits of taking HRT. First, it can improve the symptoms of hot flushes and night sweats, and most women see an improvement within the first month. Second, it can improve the symptoms of vaginal dryness and pain during sex, as well as urinary problems such as frequent urination or not being able to hold it in. Third, it offers protection against osteoporosis and so reduces the risk of fractures in the hip, spine and wrist. Finally, it reduces the risk of bowel cancer by one-third.
>
> There is uncertainty as to whether HRT also reduces the risk of heart disease and stroke and whether it delays or reduces the risk of Alzheimer disease, but these are areas being researched.

5. Common questions and sample answers include:

Q: I've heard that there's a risk of cancer with HRT. Is this true?

A: With combined HRT, there is an increased risk of breast cancer that is similar to the increased risk with a late natural menopause, which is small (2.3% increased risk per year). Once HRT is stopped for 5 years, the risk returns to that if you'd never had HRT.

With oestrogen-only HRT, there is an increased risk of endometrial cancer that increases with prolonged use and remains >5 years after stopping. There is no increased risk with continuous combined HRT, and so oestrogen-only HRT is usually only prescribed for women who have had a hysterectomy.

Other increased risks with HRT include blood clots and gallbladder disease but, in all of these cases, the absolute risks remain low.

Q: For how long do I continue HRT?

A: HRT is usually continued for 5 years, with a break and evaluation of symptoms at that time. If you suffer from osteoporosis, treatment may need to be for longer, but other agents are also available, and so a discussion as to the most appropriate management plan would need to take place at that time.

Q: I'm not comfortable with the possible effects of taking HRT. Are there any alternatives to manage my symptoms?

A: Alternatives are available for the different indications for HRT.

For hot flushes and night sweats, drugs such as fluoxetine, citalopram and venlafaxine can be effective, as may gabapentin or clonidine, though the evidence is limited.

For vaginal dryness, vitamin E oil, lubricants and moisturizers without oestrogen are available, though are less effective; topical oestrogen is not usually absorbed in significant doses, so systemic side effects do not tend to occur.

For osteoporosis, the first-line treatment is with bisphosphonates together with calcium and vitamin D; other options include strontium, raloxifene and parathyroid hormone.

Alternative therapies are also available and include soya and chickpeas, which contain natural phytoestrogens, black cohosh, evening primrose oil and others.

6. Most units will have a leaflet covering the important points of the consultation and offering advice for further support groups and counselling; it is important to give the patient one of these before she leaves.

7. Before closing the consultation, briefly summarize the discussion, check that the patient has understood and offer her a chance to ask any more questions.

BIMANUAL EXAMINATION

Score Sheet

Scores: 1 = Not attempted; 2 = Attempted, unsatisfactory; 3 = Attempted, satisfactory

Action	1	2	3
1. **W**ashes hands, **i**ntroduces self to patient, checks patient **i**dentity, explains procedure to patient and obtains **p**ermission, **p**ositions and **e**xposes patient appropriately (WIIPPE) and obtains chaperone			
2. Performs abdominal inspection, palpation and percussion			

Continued

Action	1	2	3
3. Inspects vulva and labia and comments on any abnormalities			
4. Performs bimanual vaginal examination, commenting on the vaginal wall, cervix, uterus and adnexae			
5. Disposes of clinical waste, washes hands and allows patient to dress in privacy			
6. Summarizes and presents findings to examiner			
Overall score	/18		

1. All clinical examinations should begin with these simple checks. Given the intimate nature of this examination, it is particularly important to explain to the patient what is going to happen at each step of the examination. An example would be:

   I need to perform an internal examination to check if your womb and ovaries feel healthy. This will involve me first examining your tummy by pushing gently, then inserting two gloved fingers into the vagina. I will then feel for the neck of the womb and both ovaries internally, while pushing down with the other hand on your tummy. This may be uncomfortable but shouldn't hurt. You can ask me to stop the examination at any time.

   The appropriate exposure is nude from the waist down, and it is important to tell the patient that you will leave the room/curtain area to allow her to undress and provide a sheet that she can cover herself with for when you return with a chaperone. It is also good practice to ask the patient to empty her bladder, as a full bladder interferes with the examination.

   The ideal position is lying flat on the couch. When it is time to proceed with the bimanual examination, ask the patient to bring her heels up towards her bottom and allow her knees to fall apart.

   Due to the intimate nature of the examination, a **chaperone is mandatory**.

   Remember finally that you should never perform a bimanual examination on a pregnant patient without discussing it with a senior.

2. Before proceeding with the bimanual examination, examine the abdomen as per the abdominal exam for any tenderness and masses. Start by asking the patient whether she has had/currently has any abdominal pain, then proceed with inspection for abnormalities such as lumps, scars and erythema. Next, move onto palpation, first palpating softly in the nine abdominal areas, then moving on to deep palpation. Focus particularly on the lower abdomen for masses or tenderness in the left and right iliac fossae, which may be due to ovarian pathology and, in the suprapubic region, which may be due to uterine pathology. Finally,

auscultate for bowel sounds, as obstruction may present with left or right iliac fossa pain.

3. Before exposing the patient, remember to adjust the light and wear a pair of gloves (after checking for a latex allergy).

Begin by inspecting the vulva for masses (cysts, tumours or abscesses) and infection (erythema, inflammation, ulceration or warts) and ask the patient to cough to inspect for prolapse of the pelvic organs.

Pelvic organ prolapse is where the pelvic organs descend from their physiological position due to weakness of the pelvic ligaments (the transverse cervical and uterosacral ligaments) and the pelvic floor (levator ani muscle). There are several different types, and symptoms depend on the type and extent of prolapse:

Type of prolapse	Description	Symptoms
Uterine	Prolapse of the uterus into the vagina First degree: cervix remains in the vagina Second degree: cervix descends to the introitus Third degree: entire uterus comes out of the vagina Often accompanied by vaginal vault prolapse	Heaviness/dragging sensation Impaired sexual function
Cystocele	Prolapse of the bladder, causing a bulge in the anterior vaginal wall Often accompanied by urethrocoele, a bulging of the urethra into the lower anterior vaginal wall	Urinary frequency, urgency, incomplete bladder emptying and incontinence
Rectocele	Prolapse of the rectum, causing a bulge in the posterior vaginal wall Often accompanied by enterocoele, a bulging of the pouch of Douglas into the upper posterior vaginal wall	Often asymptomatic, may cause constipation

4. Put some lubricant jelly on the index and middle fingers of your dominant hand; warn the patient that you are about to begin the internal exam. Part the labia with your non-dominant hand and insert the lubricated index and middle fingers with the palmar surface pointing medially, then turn the fingers through 90° so that the palmar surface points upwards, allowing you to bimanually ballot the uterus.

The bimanual examination should examine each of the vagina, cervix, uterus and adnexae in turn:

a. **Vagina:** Assess for any tenderness or masses (including prolapse) and note the nature of any masses as for any lump

b. **Cervix:** Assess for position (anterior or posterior), tenderness (which is known as cervical excitation) or masses and note the nature of any masses as for any lump. Note also whether the external os admits a finger (which is commonly the case with a multiparous woman)

c. **Uterus:** Employ the external hand to ballot the uterus between the fingertips of both hands, one resting on the cervix, the other on the suprapubic area. Assess for:

   i. **Size:** the uterus may be enlarged with pregnancy, fibroids or endometrial cancer

   ii. **Masses:** a smooth, regular mass or multiple masses may indicate fibroids; a rough, irregular mass may indicate a carcinoma

   iii. **Tenderness:** tenderness may indicate infection, such as pelvic inflammatory disease or endometritis

   iv. **Position:** anteverted or retroverted

   v. **Mobility:** immobility may indicate endometriosis

d. **Adnexa:** Palpate the left and right adnexa in turn by moving the internal fingers into the fornices and matching them with the external fingers over the left and right iliac fossa. Assess for the following:

   i. **Ovaries:** if you can feel an enlarged ovary or ovarian mass, it could indicate an ovarian cyst or carcinoma

   ii. **Fallopian tubes:** the fallopian tubes are normally impalpable, and tenderness could indicate salpingitis

Remove your fingers in the same way as they were inserted, and inspect the glove for signs of blood or abnormal discharge and comment appropriately.

Gynaecological tumours may be benign or malignant and may present with a pelvic mass, pain, vaginal bleeding, symptoms related to metastatic spread or the systemic effects of the disease. Further investigation of any mass appreciated during clinical examination is always necessary before making a diagnosis, but in an OSCE you should be able to present a sensible differential diagnosis based upon the examination findings:

Diagnosis	History	Examination
Uterine masses: benign		
Uterine fibroid (leiomyoma)	Most commonly asymptomatic May present with menorrhagia, dysmenorrhoea or local pressure effects, e.g. urinary retention	Either single palpable hard mass continuous with the uterus or 'lumpy/knobbly' enlargement of the uterus
Uterine tumours: malignant		
Endometrial carcinoma	Most commonly post-menopausal bleeding (PMB) Less common in younger patients, who tend to present with intermenstrual bleeding (IMB) or new-onset menorrhagia	Usually normal

Continued

Diagnosis	History	Examination
Uterine sarcoma	Leiomyosarcomas (malignant fibroids) usually present with rapid, painful enlargement of a fibroid; other sarcomas usually present with IMB or post-coital bleeding (PCB)	May have appreciable pelvic mass, particularly in the case of leiomyosarcomas

Cervical masses: malignant

Diagnosis	History	Examination
Cervical carcinoma	May be asymptomatic and diagnosed from biopsy/large loop excision of the transformation zone (LLETZ) following cervical screening and colposcopy Early disease may present with PCB, IMB, PMB or offensive vaginal discharge Late disease may present with haematuria, rectal bleeding or pain on a background of missed smears	May be normal in early disease (though will be visible at colposcopy with acetic acid staining) May have visible/palpable mass arising from the cervix that can bleed when provoked

Ovarian masses: benign

Diagnosis	History	Examination
Endometriotic 'chocolate' cyst	Rupture leads to acute pelvic pain Coexisting symptoms of endometriosis may be present	May be normal May have appreciable unilateral pelvic/adnexal mass
Benign neoplasms and functional cysts	There are a number of benign ovarian neoplasms that fall into three main groups: epithelial, germ cell and sex cord tumours. A functional cyst is a persistently enlarged follicle or corpus luteum, and so is present in pre-menopausal women only They may be asymptomatic, present with acute or chronic abdominal pain (including deep dyspareunia) or abnormal vaginal bleeding	May be normal May have appreciable unilateral or bilateral pelvic/adnexal masses Fibromas are a type of sex cord tumour that can present with Meig syndrome: ascites and a (usually) right-sided pleural effusion

Ovarian masses: malignant

Diagnosis	History	Examination
Ovarian carcinoma	90% are epithelial carcinomas and present in women over 50, more common with advanced age Classically present late with stage 3–4 disease with abdominal mass/distension/'bloating', abnormal vaginal bleeding, pain, symptoms from local compression (urinary retention/change in bowel habit) or symptoms from metastases (bowel/breast/liver/lungs)	Usually presents with late disease: unilateral or bilateral abdominal mass/distension, ascites, cachexia and/or examination findings from metastases

Continued

Diagnosis	History	Examination
Vulval/vaginal masses: benign		
Bartholin's gland cyst/ abscess	Asymptomatic or painful, particularly while sitting/walking/intercourse	Cyst or tender red swelling (abscess) in the 5 or 7 o'clock position behind the labia minora
Vaginal cyst	Asymptomatic or dyspareunia	Usually smooth, white cyst of variable size
Vulval/vaginal masses: malignant		
Vulval/vaginal carcinoma	Both usually present in older women (>60), with pruritis, bleeding, abnormal discharge or self-discovery of a mass	Visible/palpable mass or ulcer on the vulva/vagina Vaginal carcinoma is commonly a secondary from a cervical/ endometrial/vulval primary

5. Remove the gloves and dispose of them appropriately, wash your hands and allow the patient to dress in privacy.

6. An example of a summary of a normal bimanual exam is as follows:

I was asked to perform a bimanual vaginal examination on Mrs T, a 46-year-old woman who is G2P2. The abdomen was soft and non-tender, with no obvious masses felt. On inspection, the vulva and labia appeared normal with no obvious masses, inflammation or pelvic organ prolapse. On palpation, the labia and vaginal wall contained no masses or areas of tenderness. The cervix was anterior, admitted one finger into the external os and contained no masses, and there was no cervical excitation present. The uterus was balloted bimanually and was noted to be of normal size, anteverted, mobile, with no palpable masses or tenderness. Both adnexae were normal with no masses or tenderness. On removal of the hand, the glove contained no blood or abnormal discharge.

In summary the findings of the bimanual vaginal examination were a normal vulva, vagina, cervix, uterus and adnexae. To complete the examination, I would perform a speculum examination to visualize the vaginal walls and cervix directly.

SPECULUM EXAMINATION AND CERVICAL SMEAR

The speculum examination is a standard part of the examination of many presenting complaints in obstetrics and gynaecology, including vaginal bleeding, vaginal discharge, abdominal pain in pregnancy and fitting intrauterine devices. In an OSCE scenario, the speculum examination is commonly tested as part of taking a cervical smear to detect cervical intraepithelial neoplasia (CIN). An important aspect of this station is making sure that the woman is comfortable and understands fully why and how the smear will be done.

Score Sheet

Scores: 1 = Not attempted; 2 = Attempted, unsatisfactory; 3 = Attempted, satisfactory

Action	1	2	3
1. **W**ashes hands, **i**ntroduces self to patient, checks patient **i**dentity, explains **p**rocedure to patient and obtains **p**ermission, **p**ositions and **e**xposes patient appropriately (WIIPPE) and obtains a chaperone			
2. Prepares the equipment required for the examination and positions the light appropriately			
3. Inspects the vulva and comments on the findings			
4. Inserts the speculum into the vagina using an appropriate technique, visualizes the cervix and comments on the findings			
5. Introduces the brush into the external os and obtains a sample using an appropriate method			
6. Removes the speculum using an appropriate technique			
7. Thanks the patient, allows her to dress in privacy and then presents findings to the examiner			
Overall score		/21	

1. All clinical examinations should begin with these simple checks and, in this station, explaining the procedure and obtaining permission are key parts. It is important to explain to the woman why she is there and exactly what you are going to do at each step, showing her the speculum and brush that you will be using. An example might be:

> *You've been asked to come in today to have a cervical smear test. The aim of the cervical screening is not to diagnose cervical cancer but to detect any changes in the cervix, which is the neck of the womb. Most women will have normal cells, but in 1 in 20 women the test will show changes in the cells of the cervix, though most of these changes will not lead to cancer. However, if cells suggestive of pre-cancerous changes are detected, they can be removed before cervical cancer develops.*
>
> *The test will involve me passing this speculum into the vagina and taking a sample of cells from your cervix using a small brush. This may be uncomfortable but shouldn't hurt. You can ask me to stop the examination at any time.*
>
> *Once the examination is complete, you can get dressed and go home, and we will contact you with the results of the test in 2 weeks. Do you have any questions, or are you happy for me to proceed?*

Remember that a 25-year-old nulliparous woman having her first speculum and cervical smear will be much more apprehensive about such an examination than a 50-year-old multiparous woman. You should therefore adapt your approach accordingly, ensuring that you have adequately addressed the patient's concerns in order to obtain her consent.

The appropriate exposure is nude from the waist down, and it is important to tell the patient that you will leave the room/curtain area to allow her to undress and will provide a sheet that she can cover herself with for when you return with a chaperone. It is also good practice to ask the patient to empty her bladder prior to the examination.

The ideal position is lying flat on the couch. When it is time to proceed with the examination, ask the patient to bring her heels up towards her bottom and allow her knees to fall apart.

Due to the intimate nature of the examination, a **chaperone is mandatory** and you will also require her assistance while taking the cervical smear.

2. The list of equipment you will need is:

Sterile gloves	For handling the speculum, swabs, brush
Cusco's speculum	Appropriately sized for patient
Lubricating jelly	To aid with insertion of speculum
Cervical smear brush and fixative medium	To sample cervical cells
Tissue	To allow the patient to clean up after the examination

3. Before proceeding with the speculum, inspect the vulva and introitus for any masses, warts, cysts, erythema or inflammation and note the nature of any discharge.

4. Lubricate the speculum by applying jelly just below the tips of the blades (to avoid contaminating the cervix with jelly) and, before starting, ensure the patient is ready and ask her to relax as much as she can. Using your non-dominant hand part the labia; then, using your dominant hand insert the speculum gently, with the tips in the vertical orientation. As you progress the speculum, rotate it through 90° so that the handle is anterior, and then gently open the blades to bring the cervix into view. If the cervix is not seen, it may be helpful to ask the patient to place her hands beneath her buttocks to bring an anteverted cervix into view, or to ask the patient to bring her knees up to her abdomen to bring a retroverted cervix into view. Once the cervix has been visualized, you can lock the blades in position using the screw on the speculum and comment on any ectropions/erosions, polyps, bleeding, discharge or obvious masses.

5. The main method of sampling cervical cells in use in the UK is called liquid-based cytology (LBC) and involves using a plastic brush to collect

the sample, which is then transferred to a fixative solution. With the cervix in view, insert the central bristles of the brush into the endocervical canal, allowing the outer bristles to sample the ectocervix. Rotate the brush five times in a clockwise direction, applying pressure equivalent to using a pencil, and then remove the brush. Check the expiry date of the fixative vial, then insert the brush into the vial, snap off the head and screw the lid on.

There are different systems in use in different hospitals that may require slightly different techniques, so you should check the correct approach for the system you will be examined on.

6. Unlock the blades if necessary and remove the speculum gently, allowing the blades to close under pressure from the vaginal walls and rotating the speculum back through 90° to remove it in the same orientation as it was introduced.

7. Tell the patient that the examination is finished. Advise her that the results will be available in 2 weeks and that hospital will contact her to let her know whether the result was 'normal' or 'abnormal', where 'abnormal' may mean that the sample was inadequate and needs to be repeated. Advise her that it is normal to experience some spotting for the next few days, and allow her to dress in privacy. Label the sample and dispose of the used equipment appropriately.

An example of a presentation of a normal examination would be:

> *I was asked to perform a speculum examination and cervical smear test on Mrs Q, a 33-year-old woman who has come in as part of the NHS Cervical Screening Programme. On inspection, the vulva and vagina were normal, with no masses or signs of inflammation. The cervix was visualized, and there were no ectropions, polyps or masses present; there was no abnormal discharge or bleeding. The cervix was sampled using a Cervex-Brush with five clockwise rotations and fixed in an LBC vial. There was no bleeding noted, the speculum was removed and the patient was advised that she may experience some light spotting over the next few days and that the results will be available in approximately 2 weeks. In summary, this was an examination of a normal vulva, vagina and cervix, and a cervical smear was taken using a Cervex-Brush that was sent for LBC.*
>
> *To complete the examination, I would explain the possible results and follow-up to the patient and ensure that any questions or concerns that she had were addressed.*

Clinical scenario: follow-up of cervical screening

The prevalence of cervical cancer is increasing in the population, and it is the major gynaecological cancer affecting young women with a peak incidence of CIN3 in the 25- to 29-year-old age group. There is an identified necessary precursor lesion (CIN) that can be detected and treated; therefore, cervical cancer is particularly amenable to screening. This has been carried out by the NHS Cervical Screening Programme since the 1980s, reducing mortality by 50%. In clinical practice, you are most likely to encounter cervical cancer or CIN as part of cervical screening, and in an OSCE, it may come up as a discussion with a patient who has been recalled following her cervical smear or as a discussion with an examiner of how you would manage an abnormal result.

The possible results are:

Result	Explanation	Action
Normal/ negative	No dyskaryosis seen	Inform patient of normal result Investigate and manage incidental findings, e.g. infections Routine recall
Inadequate (~9% of samples)	Sample was inadequate, e.g. due to insufficient or unsuitable material, inadequate fixation or infection	If signs of infection, treat and repeat sample within 3 months If no signs of infection, repeat sample as soon as possible If three inadequate samples, advise colposcopy
Borderline nuclear abnormality (~5% of samples)	There is doubt as to whether the changes seen reflect true dyskaryosis Most women have ensuing samples that revert to normal	Repeat sample in 6 months, with three consecutive negative results 6 months apart required before returning to routine recall If borderline changes persist for three results, refer to colposcopy
Mild dyskaryosis (~5% of samples)	Nuclear abnormalities reflecting probable CIN1 (low grade) Most women have ensuing samples that return to normal	Ideally refer for colposcopy but can repeat sample in 6 months, with three consecutive negative results 6 months apart required before returning to routine recall If changes persist on two occasions, refer for colposcopy If result follows treatment for CIN2 or worse, refer for colposcopy immediately
Moderate dyskaryosis (1% of samples)	Nuclear abnormalities reflecting probable CIN2	Refer for colposcopy
Severe dyskaryosis (~0.5% of samples)	Nuclear abnormalities reflecting probable CIN3	Refer for colposcopy
Severe dyskaryosis ?invasive carcinoma (<0.1% of samples)	Nuclear and cellular abnormalities indicating probable CIN3 with additional features suggesting possibility of invasive cancer	Urgent referral to gynaecological oncologist for colposcopy

Continued

Result	Explanation	Action
(?)Glandular neoplasia	Dyskaryotic glandular cells that may represent cervical, endometrial or extra-endometrial adenocarcinoma	Urgent referral to gynaecological oncologist for colposcopy

Questions

1. What is the aetiology of cervical cancer?

   Oncogenic subtypes of human papillomavirus (HPV) account for virtually all cervical cancer diagnoses. The majority are caused by types 16 and 18, though types 31 and 33 are also oncogenic. There is a national programme to vaccinate girls aged 12–13 against HPV because it should be administered before first sexual contact. The current vaccine used in the UK and the US is Gardasil, which vaccinates against subtypes 16 and 18, which are responsible for more than 70% of cervical cancers in the UK, as well as subtypes 6 and 11, which are responsible for around 90% of genital warts.

2. What is the difference between dyskaryosis and dysplasia in the diagnosis of pre-malignancy or malignancy of the cervix?

   Cervical smears obtain a superficial sample of cells from the cervix, and the LBC test looks at the nuclei of the cells to identify cytological/cellular abnormalities that are marked as degrees of dyskaryosis. Although the level of dyskaryosis does, in part, reflect the severity of CIN, the grade of CIN is a histological diagnosis that must be made on a tissue sample from biopsy at colposcopy. With a biopsy sample, it is possible to see whether the atypical cells are only in the lower third of the epithelium (CIN1) or in the lower two-thirds (CIN2) or if they occupy the full thickness of the epithelium (CIN3).

3. Following cervical screening, what are the indications for colposcopy?

   The indications for colposcopy include:
   a. Single smear showing moderate or severe dyskaryosis
   b. Single smear suggestive of invasive carcinoma or glandular neoplasia
   c. Single smear or two consecutive smears showing mild dyskaryosis depending on local protocols
   d. Three consecutive borderline or inadequate smears
   e. Abnormal looking cervix

4. What are the key steps of colposcopy?

   The key steps of colposcopy include:
   a. Inspection of the transformation zone (TZ) of the cervix under microscopy
   b. Staining of the TZ with 5% acetic acid or Lugol's iodine

    c. Punch biopsy of the abnormal area, or 'see and treat' with large loop excision of the transformation zone (LLETZ), followed by sending the sample for biopsy to ensure adequate margins

5. Other than through cervical screening, how else might a patient with cervical cancer present?

Established cervical cancer can present with abnormal vaginal bleeding, e.g. post-coital bleeding, intermenstrual bleeding or post-menopausal bleeding. In advanced disease, involvement of local structures may lead to haematuria, rectal bleeding and pain. A history of missed cervical smear tests is common.

BREAKING BAD NEWS

Case 1: ectopic pregnancy

'You are an FY1 doctor in obstetrics and gynaecology. Mrs E, a 26-year-old woman, has presented to the early pregnancy assessment unit with a small amount of vaginal bleeding and some mild colicky left iliac fossa pain, both of which have now stopped. She had a positive pregnancy test 4 weeks ago, which has been confirmed today, and she is 8+4 weeks' pregnant by her last menstrual period. She has been clerked by the specialist nurse and has no risk factors for ectopic pregnancy. Abdominal examination was normal. A transvaginal ultrasound scan has been performed and confirms an ectopic pregnancy in the left fallopian tube. Explain these findings to the patient, discuss the next steps in management and counsel her appropriately.'

Score Sheet

Scores: 1 = Not attempted; 2 = Attempted, unsatisfactory; 3 = Attempted, satisfactory

Action	1	2	3
1. Introduces self, checks patient's name, date of birth and occupation and develops rapport			
2. Clarifies history of presenting complaint			
3. Establishes what the patient has been told already about the ultrasound scan and sensitively breaks bad news using simple terms			
4. Answers typical questions appropriately			
5. Discusses options for management with the patient			
6. Provides leaflets with further information and support groups			
7. Summarizes and closes consultation appropriately			
Overall score		/21	

1. Start any consultation with a patient by introducing yourself and making sure that you are seeing the correct patient by checking patient's name and date of birth. Checking patient's occupation gives you additional

information, such as how much prior understanding she may have of the diagnosis and how much time she may need off work. This also helps to build rapport, which is particularly important in this sort of scenario.

2. In a discussion or breaking bad news station, it is likely that you will be provided with all of the important details from the history and examination so that you do not have to repeat this process, as is the case here. However, recapping the history will better place you to be able to explain the findings and will also help to build rapport. This can be done quickly, e.g.:

> *I understand that you're about 8-and a-half weeks pregnant, and you've come into hospital with a small amount of vaginal bleeding and some mild pain in the bottom left of your abdomen; is that correct? Have you had any other symptoms at all?*

3. In order to break bad news appropriately, it is important to gauge how much the patient already knows. Ultrasound scans are performed with the woman awake, obviously concerned about her symptoms and/or her pregnancy and, so, the ultrasonographers are commonly asked for information at the time of the scan. A simple question will elicit whether she has been told the result already and you can modify your explanation accordingly:

> *I can see that you've had an ultrasound scan; has anybody spoken to you about the results yet? And what have they told you?*

Breaking bad news sensitively is about what you say (use simple, clear language, listen and respond empathetically), how you say it (speak slowly, with appropriate pauses), your body language (keep an open posture and nod your head to reassure her that you are listening to her concerns) and eye contact. Use pauses and silences to give the patient a chance to digest significant pieces of information and to ask questions; never interrupt. An example of how you might explain the finding of an ectopic pregnancy to a patient would be:

> *I have your ultrasound report, and I'm afraid I have to give you some difficult news. The ultrasound shows that your pregnancy is growing outside of the uterus, in your left fallopian tube. This is what is known as an ectopic pregnancy, and it is likely to be the reason that you have been having vaginal bleeding and lower abdominal pain. Unfortunately, ectopic pregnancies are not viable and can be very dangerous to your health and will have to be removed.*
>
> *Do you have any questions before we discuss what happens next?*

4. Common questions and sample answers include:

Q: Why did this happen? Was it something I did wrong?

A: This isn't your fault, and there was nothing that you could have done to prevent it from happening, so you mustn't blame yourself. About 1 in 100 pregnancies are ectopic, and in more than half the cases, we don't know why it happened. The risk factors that we do know about are previous infection or surgery close to the fallopian tubes, assisted conception such as IVF and a condition called endometriosis. Smoking has also been linked to an increased risk of ectopic pregnancy.

Q: Will it happen again?

A: The risk of recurrence is between 10% and 20%, so it is higher than in women who have not had an ectopic pregnancy; however, the majority of women who have had an ectopic pregnancy go on to conceive normally. The next time you become pregnant, we would advise you to see your GP to have an early ultrasound to determine the location of the pregnancy.

Q: Why does it have to be removed; can it not just grow where it is?

A: The fallopian tubes are much smaller than the uterus and are not designed to stretch and grow in the same way that the uterus is. Unfortunately, that means that, if the pregnancy continued to grow in the fallopian tube, it is at risk of rupturing, which can cause a lot of bleeding and is ultimately a life-threatening event. For this reason, it is very important that it is removed and we can talk through the options now.

5. There are three management options:

a. **Surgery**: The preferred method of management is to admit the patient directly for surgical management because it removes the risk of rupture straight away. The ideal procedure is a laparoscopic salpingectomy (removal of ectopic pregnancy and fallopian tube) because this carries the lowest risk to the patient and prevents recurrence in the same tube. In an emergency, e.g. a haemodynamically unstable patient with a ruptured ectopic pregnancy, a laparotomy may be necessary, and if the woman has already had one fallopian tube removed or the other tube is visibly diseased/damaged, then a salpingotomy would be more appropriate (removal of ectopic pregnancy with retention of the fallopian tube).

The other two options of expectant management (watch and wait) and methotrexate are only available if strict criteria are met, notably:

i. Clinically stable and minimal symptoms

ii. Low hCG level (<3000 IU)

iii. Small ectopic pregnancy (<3 cm)

iv. Fully understands the signs and symptoms and implications of ectopic pregnancy and the possibility of rupture at any time (with written information provided) and lives close enough to hospital with support at home

In these cases, the other two options are:

b. **Methotrexate:** If the above (or local) criteria have been met, the patient can be considered for methotrexate, which is administered as an intramuscular injection, followed by hCG levels on days 4 and 7, followed by a second dose if the fall in hCG from day 4 to day 7 is <15%. Side effects include conjunctivitis, stomatitis (inflammation of the mucous lining of the mouth) and GI symptoms, including abdominal pain.

c. **Expectant:** If the above (or local) criteria have been met, the patient can be considered for expectant management, which is watchful waiting while taking serial 48-hour hCG levels until falling, then weekly hCG levels until <15 IU.

You should counsel the woman regarding all three options if appropriate, while advising her that the safest course of action is laparoscopic surgery. Remember that if the patient is well and stable, she may want to discuss it with her partner or family before making a decision.

6. Most units will have a leaflet covering the important points of the consultation, offering advice for further support groups and counselling; it is important to give the patient one of these before she leaves. This is particularly the case if she is not being admitted for surgery and is going home with medical/expectant management.

7. Before closing the consultation, briefly summarize the discussion, check that the patient has understood and offer her a chance to ask any more questions.

Case 2: miscarriage

'You are an FY1 doctor in obstetrics and gynaecology. Mrs E, a 32-year-old woman, has presented to the early pregnancy assessment unit with a single episode of vaginal bleeding associated with ongoing cramping lower abdominal pain. She had a positive pregnancy test 4 weeks ago, which has been confirmed today, and she is 7+0 weeks pregnant by her last menstrual period. A transvaginal ultrasound scan has been performed and confirms an incomplete miscarriage, with an empty gestational sac seen. Explain these findings to the patient, discuss the next steps in management and counsel her appropriately.'

Score Sheet

Scores: 1 = Not attempted; 2 = Attempted, unsatisfactory; 3 = Attempted, satisfactory

Action	1	2	3
1. Introduces self, checks patient's name, date of birth and occupation and develops rapport			
2. Clarifies history of presenting complaint			

Continued

Action	1	2	3
3. Establishes what the patient has been told already about the ultrasound scan and sensitively breaks bad news using simple terms			
4. Answers typical questions appropriately			
5. Discusses options for management with the patient			
6. Provides leaflets with further information and support groups			
7. Summarizes and closes consultation appropriately			
Overall score	/21		

1. Start any consultation with a patient by introducing yourself and making sure that you are seeing the correct patient by checking patient's name and date of birth. Checking patient's occupation gives you additional information, such as how much prior understanding she may have of the diagnosis and how much time she may need off work. This also helps to build rapport, which is particularly important in this sort of scenario.

2. In a discussion or breaking bad news station, it is likely that you will be provided with all of the important details from the history and examination so that you do not have to repeat this process, as is the case here. However, recapping the history will better place you to be able to explain the findings and will also help to build rapport. This can be done quickly, e.g.:

   > *I understand that you've come into hospital with some vaginal bleeding and cramping abdominal pain, with a positive pregnancy test; is that correct? And have you had any other symptoms at all?*

3. In order to break bad news appropriately, it is important to gauge how much the patient already knows. Ultrasound scans are performed with the woman awake, obviously concerned about her symptoms and/or her pregnancy and, so, the ultrasonographers are commonly asked for information at the time of the scan. A simple question will elicit whether she has been told the result already and you can modify your explanation accordingly:

   > *I can see that you've had an ultrasound scan; has anybody spoken to you about the results yet? And what have they told you?*

   Breaking bad news sensitively is about what you say (use simple, clear language, listen and respond empathetically), how you say it (speak slowly, with appropriate pauses), your body language (keep an open posture and nod your head to reassure her that you are listening to her concerns) and eye contact. Use pauses and silences to give the patient a chance to digest significant pieces of information and to ask questions; never interrupt.

An example of how you might explain the finding of an incomplete miscarriage to a patient would be:

> *I have your ultrasound report, and I'm afraid I have to give you some difficult news. The ultrasound shows that you are having a miscarriage and that is likely to be causing your bleeding and pain. I'm very sorry.*
>
> *Unfortunately miscarriages occur in around 10%–20% of pregnancies; in most cases, we don't know why it happens and nothing you did or didn't do is likely to have caused the miscarriage.*
>
> *Do you have any questions before we discuss what happens next?*

4. Common questions and sample answers include:

Q: Why did this happen? Was it something I did wrong?

A: In most cases we don't know why a miscarriage occurs. It is thought that most miscarriages are caused by a one-off genetic fault that means that the fetus is unable to grow and develop and, so, the pregnancy ends with a miscarriage. Less commonly, miscarriages can be caused by hormonal imbalances or infections. It is unlikely that anything you did or didn't do caused the miscarriage; in particular, lifting, straining, stress, sexual intercourse or exercise do not cause miscarriages. Things that increase the risk of miscarriage include your age, drug and alcohol abuse, smoking and poorly controlled disease such as diabetes.

Q: If it happened this time, does that mean that it will happen again?

A: The vast majority of women who have a miscarriage go on to have a successful pregnancy. Recurrent miscarriages, where there are three miscarriages in a row, happen in around 1% of women and, in these cases, we undertake further tests to see if there is an underlying cause.

Q: Is there anything we could have done to stop it?

A: Unfortunately, there is nothing that could have been done to stop it because there is no treatment to prevent a miscarriage.

Q: When will we be able to try for a baby again?

A: You can try again after your next period, which may take a little longer to come, but the best time is when you and your partner feel both physically and emotionally ready.

5. There are three management options:

a. **Surgery:** Surgical management is by evacuation of retained products of conception (ERPC), which is a slightly different procedure than dilation and curettage (D&C), which involves sharp curettage. ERPC is carried out using suction curettage under general or local anaesthesia, though the latter is rarely conducted in the UK. The Royal College of Obstetricians and Gynaecologists (RCOG) guidelines advise that it should be offered to all women to decide based on preference, but clear indications include: persistent excessive bleeding, haemodynamic instability, evidence of infected retained tissue or suspected gestational trophoblastic disease.

The complications include: heavy bleeding, infection, incomplete evacuation requiring repeat procedure and, rarely, uterine perforation requiring laparoscopic or open repair.

b. **Medical:** Medical management is possible using prostaglandin analogues (gemeprost or misoprostol), which may be given orally or vaginally, with or without an antiprogesterone (mifepristone) depending on local protocols. RCOG guidelines note that efficacy varies widely from 13% to 96%, influenced by type of miscarriage, sac size and whether follow-up is clinical or by ultrasound.

Patients should be warned that, if effective, the medication takes a few hours to take effect, at which point they will experience an increase in pain and bleeding similar to a heavy period. The bleeding may continue for up to 3 weeks. If medical management is unsuccessful or incomplete, then they should be advised to proceed with surgery. Medical management may be undertaken as an inpatient or outpatient depending on the clinical situation, patient choice and local protocols.

c. **Expectant:** Expectant management is what is explained to patients as 'letting nature take its course'. It is effective, though RCOG guidelines note again that efficacy varies widely from 25% to 100%.

Patients should be warned that complete resolution can take several weeks, particularly with missed miscarriage, though normally less than 3 weeks in incomplete miscarriage. The risk of infection rises with duration for completing the miscarriage and, so, a plan should be made for when they should come back to consider medical/surgical management as per local protocols. Finally, the bleeding can be heavy and may uncommonly require emergency admission to hospital.

You should counsel the woman regarding all three options if she can access 24-hour telephone advice and emergency admission if required, while advising her that surgery always remains available if the other options fail. Remember that if the patient is well and stable, she may want to discuss it with her partner or family before making a decision.

Women who are rhesus (Rh) negative should receive anti-D if >12 weeks (all women) or <12 weeks and having medical/surgical management or heavy bleeding or severe pain.

6. Most units will have a leaflet covering the important points of the consultation, offering advice for further support groups and counselling; it is important to give the patient one of these before she leaves. The leaflet should also contain details of the ERPC and advice on when to call for help, namely:
   a. Concerning amount of bleeding
   b. Concerning amount of pain
   c. Abnormal vaginal discharge
   d. Fever, shivers or feeling systemically unwell

  e. Feeling dizzy or faint
  f. Shoulder pain
7. Before closing the consultation, briefly summarize the discussion, check that the patient has understood and offer her a chance to ask any more questions.

WHO classification of the stages of spontaneous miscarriage

Stage	Description
Threatened miscarriage (this is the only stage compatible with continued pregnancy)	Unprovoked vaginal bleeding, with or without abdominal pain, before 22 weeks' gestation. Compatible with continuing viable pregnancy.
Inevitable miscarriage	Specific clinical features (vaginal bleeding and open cervical os) indicate that the pregnancy is in the process of expulsion from the uterus. Will proceed to incomplete or complete miscarriage.
Incomplete miscarriage	Miscarriage at the stage that the products of conception are partially expelled.
Complete miscarriage	Miscarriage in which the products of conception are completely expelled.
Missed miscarriage	Ultrasound features consistent with a non-viable or non-continuing pregnancy, even in the absence of clinical features, usually as an incidental finding.

GENERAL OBSTETRIC HISTORY

Score Sheet

Scores: 1 = Not attempted; 2 = Attempted, unsatisfactory; 3 = Attempted, satisfactory

Action	1	2	3
1. Introduces self appropriately, establishes rapport and checks occupation			
2. Establishes background to current pregnancy and calculates the gestation and estimated date of delivery			
3. Elicits the patient's complaints and concerns and explores the history of each presenting complaint			
4. Enquires about any tests the patient may have had and their results			
5. Elicits a brief gynaecological history			
6. Elicits a focused past medical and surgical history			
7. Elicits a complete drug and allergy history			
8. Elicits a relevant family history			
9. Elicits the patient's social history			
10. Checks with the patient that she has no additional concerns or things she would like to discuss			
11. Summarizes and presents findings			
Overall score		/33	

1. Always begin a clinical history station by introducing yourself, establishing that the correct patient is sitting in front of you by checking patient's name, date of birth and occupation. It is also important to check the patient's relationship status to ensure that appropriate support is available to her ante-, intra- and postpartum.

2. Although the standard approach to history taking is to begin with the presenting complaint, in an obstetric history it is often useful to check the past obstetric history to better place the presenting complaint in context. This should include:

   a. **Gravidity** (total number of pregnancies, including the current one) and **parity** (number of pregnancies carried beyond 24 weeks+ losses before this time). This will normally be written as, e.g. G4 P2+1, denoting a fourth pregnancy, with two live children and one miscarriage before 24 weeks. For each pregnancy, it is important to note the gestation, outcome, mode of delivery and any complications, e.g. intrauterine growth restriction (IUGR), pre-eclampsia, gestational diabetes, shoulder dystocia or postpartum haemorrhage.

   b. Establish the date of the last menstrual period (LMP), regularity of cycle (regular or irregular) and cycle length. Calculate the estimated date of delivery (EDD) by LMP, using the formula:

   $$EDD = LMP - 3 \ months + 1 \ year + 7 \ days + (cycle \ length - 28 \ days)$$

   Alternatively, an obstetric wheel may be used. Note that, once the dating scan has taken place, the scan date tends to be used for the definitive EDD.

   c. Whether this was a **planned pregnancy**, if so whether there is any history of subfertility or assisted conception, e.g. IVF. If this is not a planned pregnancy, ask whether any **contraceptives** were used. Note particularly that the copper IUD increases the risk of ectopic pregnancy.

   d. **Rhesus status:** If the patient is rhesus positive, then no further action is required. If the patient is rhesus negative, then she will require anti-D routinely at around 30 weeks, following any sensitizing event after 12 weeks (any antenatal bleed or abdominal trauma) and will require a Kleihauer test postnatally to assess for a further dose.

   e. **Placental location** is assessed at the 20-week scan. Note particularly if there is any degree of placenta praevia (placenta covering os) or if the placenta is low.

   f. **Pregnancy-related complications**, or if the pregnancy has been uneventful so far. Ask specifically about:

      i. Vaginal bleeding, discharge or abdominal pain

      ii. Raised blood pressure, peripheral/facial oedema or diagnosed pre-eclampsia

      iii. Glycosuria, raised capillary glucose or diagnosed gestational diabetes mellitus

iv. Jaundice, itching, pale stools, dark urine or diagnosed obstetric cholestasis

v. Any diagnosed infections

For any positive findings, ask about the results of any investigations, management instituted and follow-up.

3. The presenting complaint(s) should be elicited from the patient with an open question, for example: 'What's brought you in to see us today?' Patients may have more than one presenting complaint, for example, abdominal pain and vaginal bleeding, in which case you should document each symptom in the patient's own words and take a history of presenting complaint for each. Common examples include:

Presenting complaint	History of presenting complaint
Abdominal pain	Use the 'SOCRATES' tool: **Site:** Where is the pain now and does that differ from where it was when it first started? Any epigastric or right upper quadrant (RUQ) component? **Onset:** Is the pain acute or chronic; when did it start; did it come on suddenly, over a minute or so or more gradually and what was the patient doing at the time of onset? Is there any relationship with intercourse and have there been any unwell contacts? **Character:** What is the nature of the pain (cramping, sharp, dull, burning)? Try not to put words into the patient's mouth, instead document her answer in her own words. **Radiation:** Does the pain radiate anywhere else or is it fixed in one spot? **Associated symptoms:** Any vaginal bleeding or discharge; any frontal headache, visual disturbances, flashing lights or new-onset oedema; any diarrhoea, constipation, nausea or vomiting; any urinary frequency, urgency or dysuria; or any other associated symptoms? **Timing:** Is the pain constant or intermittent; what is the frequency; are there precipitating factors or is it always there; is it getting better or worse? Any past history of similar pain? **Exacerbating and relieving factors:** Does anything make the pain better or worse; for example, is it better lying still or moving around and is it worse after eating? Has she tried using simple analgesia such as paracetamol or co-codamol? **Severity:** For example, on a score of 1–10, how bad is the pain?
Vaginal bleeding	**Onset and Timing:** When did it first start; what was the patient doing when it started (any intercourse or trauma); how long did she bleed for; has it stopped now; how often is she bleeding; any previous vaginal bleeding? **Character:** Was the bleeding small in volume (spotting) or large in volume; were there any clots; was the patient using pads or tampons or both; how often were pads or tampons being changed; did they soak through onto the patient's clothing?

1: Obstetrics and Gynaecology

53

Continued

Presenting complaint	History of presenting complaint
	Associated symptoms: Any abdominal pain; is it constant or cramping; any change in fetal movements; any vaginal discharge; any dizziness or lightheadedness; any other symptoms? For **early pregnancies** (<24 weeks), bleeding may be associated with **miscarriage, ectopic pregnancy** or **gestational trophoblastic disease.** Accordingly, it is important to ask about: previous miscarriages and risk factors for miscarriage (e.g. smoking, alcohol, illicit drug use, amniocentesis/chorionic villus sampling [CVS], hypertension, diabetes, PCOS, systemic lupus erythematosus [SLE] and certain medications), risk factors for an ectopic pregnancy (previous ectopic pregnancy, pelvic/tubal surgery, PID, IUCD, smoking, assisted conception/IVF, endometriosis) and previous history of gestational trophoblastic disease. For **late pregnancies** (>24 weeks), bleeding may be associated with **placenta praevia, placental abruption, uterine rupture, vasa praevia** or **cervical causes.** Accordingly, it is important to ask about placental location and previous uterine surgery and clarify if any risk factors for each cause are present.
Vaginal discharge	**Onset and timing:** When did it first start; is it getting better or worse; any history of similar discharge or sexually transmitted infections; any new partners; is the partner experiencing any discharge symptoms? **Character:** Colour, volume, consistency, odour, bloodstaining? **Associated symptoms:** Any abdominal pain, vaginal bleeding or itching?
Headache	**Site:** Where in the head does she feel the headache – specifically any frontal component? **Onset:** Is the headache acute or chronic? When did it start and did it come on suddenly, over a minute or so or more gradually? What was the patient doing at the time of onset and is the patient dehydrated? Have there been any unwell contacts? **Character:** Is it sharp or dull; does it feel like a band across the front of the head; a throbbing unilateral pain? **Associated symptoms:** Any epigastric or RUQ pain, visual disturbances or flashing lights, nausea, vomiting or recent onset peripheral or facial oedema? Any neck stiffness, photophobia, drowsiness or confusion? Any focal neurology? **Timing:** Is the pain constant or intermittent; what is the frequency; are there precipitating factors or is it always there; is it getting better or worse; any past history of similar pain? **Severity:** For example, on a scale of 1–10, how bad is the headache?
Itching	**Site:** Where is the itching; has it progressed since it started? **Onset and timing:** When did it start; is it there all the time or does it fluctuate; is it getting better or worse; any history of similar itching; history of gallstones? **Associated symptoms:** Any jaundice, rash, epigastric/RUQ pain, pale stools, dark urine, anorexia?

4. Ask about investigations so far, including blood tests, ultrasound, amniocentesis or CVS. The recommended schedule for investigations is as follows:

Stage	Recommended investigations (NICE guidance, 2010)
Booking, ideally before 10 weeks	Height, weight, BMI and BP Offer screening: Urine: proteinuria and asymptomatic bacteriuria Bloods: glucose, blood group, rhesus status and alloantibodies, screening for anaemia, haemoglobinopathies (sickle cell anaemia and thalassaemias), hepatitis B virus, HIV, rubella and syphilis Down syndrome screening at following appointment if patient consents
Between 10+0 and 13+6 weeks	Either (if Down syndrome screening refused): Ultrasound between 10+0 and 13+6 for crown-rump (CR) length to determine gestational age (and head circumference if CR length is above 84 mm) Or (if Down syndrome screening consented to): Combined test: ultrasound between 11+0 and 13+6 for CR length and nuchal translucency, together with serum test (β-HCG and PAPP-A)
Between 11+0 and 13+6 weeks	(If initial screening tests indicate that CVS should be offered) CVS is usually performed in this window, depending on the timing of the initial screening tests
After 15+0 weeks	(If initial screening tests indicate that amniocentesis should be offered) Amniocentesis should be performed after 15+0 weeks' gestation. Amniocentesis performed before 14+0 weeks is referred to as 'early amniocentesis' and carries a higher rate of fetal loss, fetal talipes and respiratory morbidity
Between 15+0 and 20+0 weeks	(If Down syndrome screening consented to after window for nuchal translucency scan) Triple test (β-HCG, alpha fetoprotein and unconjugated estriol) or quadruple test for Down syndrome (β-HCG, alpha fetoprotein, inhibin-A, and unconjugated estriol)
16 weeks	Review of initial blood, urine and ultrasound investigations BP, proteinuria, and further investigation and treatment of Hb <11 g/dl
Between 18+0 and 20+6	Ultrasound screening for structural abnormalities (routine anomaly scan) If placenta extends across internal cervical os, offer additional scan at 32 weeks
25 weeks (for nulliparous women only)	BP and proteinuria Measure and plot symphysis-fundal height (SFH)
28 weeks	Offer second screening for anaemia and red-cell alloantibodies Investigate and treat Hb <10.5 g/dl Offer anti-D prophylaxis to women who are rhesus-D negative (either single dose at 28–30 weeks or two doses at 28 and 34 weeks) BP, proteinuria and measure and plot SFH

Continued

Stage	Recommended investigations (NICE guidance, 2010)
31 weeks (for nulliparous women only)	Review of 28-week screening bloods BP, proteinuria and measure and plot SFH
32 weeks	(If placenta found to be covering internal os at anomaly scan) Ultrasound scan for placenta praevia
34 weeks	Review of 28-week screening bloods Offer second dose of anti-D prophylaxis to women who are rhesus-D negative (if two-dose protocol used) BP, proteinuria and measure and plot SFH
36 weeks	Check position of baby, offer external cephalic version (ECV) if breech BP, proteinuria and measure and plot SFH
38 weeks	BP, proteinuria and measure and plot SFH
40 weeks (for nulliparous women only)	BP, proteinuria and measure and plot SFH
41 weeks	Offer membrane sweep and induction of labour BP, proteinuria and measure and plot SFH
42 weeks+	Women who have not given birth by 42 weeks and decline induction should be advised of risks and offered increased monitoring including: At least twice weekly cardiotocography (CTG) Ultrasound examination of maximum amniotic pool depth

5. The **past gynaecological history** should be brief and to the point and should include:
   a. Contraception use prior to pregnancy
   b. Date of previous cervical smear and result
   c. Previous gynaecological/pelvic procedures and surgery
6. The **past medical and surgical history** should be focused and include:
   a. Any current and past medical conditions, specifically including hypertension, diabetes, epilepsy, VTE, liver disease, thalassaemias, sickle cell disease and SLE
   b. Any previous surgery, particularly abdominal or pelvic surgery, and whether under local anaesthetic or general anaesthetic
7. The drug and allergy history should include:
   a. Prescribed and over-the-counter medications, including herbal remedies
   b. Prenatal/early pregnancy folic acid
   c. Any allergies and the nature of the allergy, i.e. rash, GI disturbance, anaphylaxis
8. Complete a **family history** largely as you would in a medical history station but also checking for:
   a. Family history of pregnancy-induced hypertension, pre-eclampsia or gestational diabetes

b. History of congenital illnesses that run in the family
c. Consanguinity in the family
d. Twin births in the family

9. The **social history** should include:
   a. Smoker, ex-smoker or non-smoker, including amount smoked, when started and when stopped
   b. Alcohol intake prior to and during pregnancy
   c. Recreational drug use prior to and during pregnancy
   d. Situation at home, i.e. single, stable partner or married, any difficulties, emotional or physical abuse, named social worker, particularly with teenage pregnancies
   e. Plans for breastfeeding

10. Unlike a medical history, a full systems review is not normally part of an obstetric history. However, it is always a good idea to give the patient a final opportunity to mention any concerns that she might have and any symptoms that she might have forgotten in the initial discussion or to ask whether there is anything else she would like to discuss.

11. Summarize the positive and key negative findings back to the patient and check that the information is accurate; thank the patient and then turn to the examiner and present. An example of a presentation of a well antenatal patient at the routine 38-week check:

> *This is a 26-year-old woman, G2 P1, with a previous uncomplicated pregnancy with a normal vaginal delivery at 39 weeks of a baby boy weighing 3.5 kg. She is 38 weeks' pregnant with an estimated delivery date by ultrasound of DD/MM/YY; it is a planned pregnancy, she is rhesus positive and her placenta is anterior, not low. She has come in today for her routine 38-week check, she feels well, the baby is active and kicking and she is otherwise asymptomatic. The pregnancy has been uncomplicated so far, with no abnormalities on the booking bloods and a normal routine ultrasound at 20 weeks. Her last cervical smear was last year and was normal; before deciding to try for a second child she was using the COCP for contraception. She has no other medical conditions, has never had any surgical procedures and is only taking antenatal vitamins and minerals and took pre-conception folic acid. She has no allergies, no family history of pregnancy-related problems or congenital illnesses, has never smoked and usually drinks around a bottle of wine over the course of the week, though hasn't had any alcohol since trying for a baby. She lives with her husband and 2-year-old boy at home, and she has no further concerns.*
>
> *In summary, this is a 26-year-old woman, 38 weeks' pregnant with her second child, who is fit and well and has no concerns today. To complete the antenatal check, I would inspect and*

palpate the abdomen to assess fetal lie and presentation, measure the symphysis-fundal height, auscultate the fetal heartbeat, check the blood pressure and dip the urine for proteinuria.

DISCUSSION WITH AN EXAMINER 1: ANTEPARTUM HAEMORRHAGE

Antepartum haemorrhage (APH) refers to any vaginal bleeding after 24 weeks' gestation, at which point the fetus is said to be viable. This should be distinguished from 'bleeding in early pregnancy', which can be due to miscarriage, ectopic pregnancy or gestational trophoblastic disease and is covered in the gynaecology section. It occurs in 3%–5% of pregnancies; most commonly no underlying cause is found, and it is attributed to minor placental abruptions. Important causes include placenta praevia and placental abruption; these will require urgent management based on RCOG Green-top guidelines. In the clinical setting, patients can present with minor bleeds to their GP or the pregnancy assessment unit or with major haemorrhage to A&E or resus. In the OSCE setting, this scenario is likely to come up as a discussion with the examiner. The main presentations include:

Diagnosis	Features on history
Placenta praevia	Painless vaginal bleeding, may be intermittent bleeds increasing in frequency and severity
	Background of low-lying placenta/placenta praevia on ultrasound
Placental abruption	Sudden onset abdominal pain with vaginal bleeding, blood may be dark
	May be 'concealed' and present only with abdominal pain (or backache with posterior placenta)
	May have contractions/be in labour
	May be in hypovolaemic shock
Vasa praevia	Vasa praevia is the presence of fetal vessels in the membrane in front of the presenting part, and presents with:
	Painless vaginal bleeding following rupture of membranes (spontaneous or with amniotomy)
	Rapid severe fetal distress and usually death
Cervical causes	Cervical causes include carcinomas, ectropions and polyps and may present with or without pregnancy
	Typically present with small recurrent post-coital bleeding but a full assessment for abruption/praevia will still be necessary
Undetermined origin (minor placental abruption)	Most cases of APH present with small-volume, painless vaginal bleeding and no previous low-lying placenta/praevia on ultrasound
	These are most likely due to minor placental abruptions, and patients should be monitored to check for further abruption

Questions

1. What are the differences in findings on history and examination in placenta praevia and placental abruption?

   Typically, in placenta praevia, the patient will present with bright red vaginal bleeding, not associated with pain and, if shocked, the level of shock tends to be consistent with external loss. On examination, the uterus will be non-tender and the fetus often has an abnormal lie with a high presenting part. If the patient has had a previous ultrasound, it will have shown a low-lying placenta or placenta praevia (the 20-week scan should have been repeated at 32 weeks if the placenta is low lying). In known or suspected placenta praevia, a digital vaginal examination should not be performed prior to an ultrasound to confirm or rule out the diagnosis.

Typically in placental abruption, the patient will present with sudden onset abdominal pain, with or without vaginal bleeding, which may be dark in colour. If the patient is shocked, it may be out of proportion to external loss due to 'concealed' bleeding. On examination, the uterus will be tender or hard, and the fetus may be engaged and distressed.

2. What are the risk factors for placenta praevia and placental abruption?
   Risk factors common to both include: multiparity, assisted conception, advanced maternal age and smoking.

   Specific risk factors for placental abruption include: abruption in previous pregnancy, pre-eclampsia, IUGR, non-vertex presentations, polyhydramnios, low BMI, intrauterine infection, premature rupture of membranes, abdominal trauma, cocaine/amphetamine misuse during pregnancy and first trimester bleeding. Maternal thrombophilias may increase the risk of abruption, but the evidence is weak.

   Specific risk factors for placenta praevia include previous placenta praevia, previous caesarean section (increasing with each surgery), previous termination of pregnancy (TOP), multiple pregnancy and deficient endometrium due to presence/history of uterine scar, endometritis, manual removal of placenta, curettage or submucous fibroid.

3. What are the complications associated with APH?
   Complications from APH can be divided into maternal and fetal complications.

   Maternal complications include: hypovolaemic shock, consumptive coagulopathy, anaemia, infection, postpartum haemorrhage, renal tubular necrosis, complications of transfusion and psychological sequelae.

   Fetal complications include: small for dates/IUGR, prematurity, hypoxia and death. Due to the increased risk of prematurity, a course of corticosteroids should be offered to women presenting with APH before 34+6 weeks of pregnancy to mature the lungs.

4. What investigations are indicated in the investigation of APH?
   Both the mother and the fetus need to be investigated.

   For the maternal investigation, initial blood tests should include: FBC, coagulation screen, crossmatch (4+ units), urea and electrolytes (U&Es) and liver function tests (LFTs). In minor haemorrhage, a group and save may be appropriate in place of crossmatching four units, keeping in mind that blood loss may be concealed.

In all women who are Rh-D negative, a Kleihauer test should be performed to assess the amount of feto-maternal haemorrhage in order to give the appropriate dose of anti-D Ig, though this is not a sensitive test for abruption.

If the placental site is not already known, ultrasound can be used to confirm or rule out placenta praevia but, again, this is not a sensitive test for abruption/retroplacental clot and will only detect 25% of cases.

For fetal investigation, CTG monitoring of heart rate should be undertaken once the mother is stable or resuscitation has commenced, or if fetal heart rate cannot be detected, then ultrasound detection of fetal heart pulsation should be undertaken.

5. When should women with APH be delivered?
   In the case of fetal death, most women should be delivered, once stable, by vaginal delivery but some may require caesarean section.

   In the case of maternal and/or fetal compromise, the woman should be resuscitated concurrent with delivery by 'emergency' caesarean section.

   In the case of no maternal or fetal compromise, there is no clear guidance and decisions regarding time, and mode of delivery should be taken by a senior obstetrician.

6. When would you discharge a patient with a minor APH of undetermined origin?
   If the woman presented with 'spotting' and an uncomplicated obstetric history, the bleeding has stopped and the initial maternal and fetal investigations are reassuring, then she can be discharged directly. If the woman presented with APH any heavier than 'spotting', or the bleeding is ongoing, then she should be admitted for further observation, with discharge to be planned after review by a senior obstetrician. Each woman should be assessed on an individual basis and, if there is any cause for concern, e.g. a past obstetric history of abruption, she should be admitted for observation.

DISCUSSION WITH AN EXAMINER 2: PRE-ECLAMPSIA

Pre-eclampsia is a multisystem disorder of placental origin that usually presents with hypertension and proteinuria (though it can affect any organ) and is a major cause of maternal morbidity and mortality. It may present with only mild hypertension and proteinuria at term, or it may present with early-onset severe hypertension, proteinuria and life-threatening complications such as an eclamptic seizure. Accordingly, it is important to have a thorough understanding of the assessment and management of pre-eclampsia, which are based upon NICE guidelines. Because the presentation is so variable, in clinical practice you could encounter pre-eclampsia in general practice, a routine antenatal appointment,

the pregnancy 'day assessment unit' or A&E/resus. In the OSCE setting, you are likely to encounter this topic as a discussion with an examiner.

Questions

1. What are the different ways in which hypertension can present in pregnancy?

   Most hypertensive disorders in pregnancy present in the second half of pregnancy, and there are three main types:
   a. Gestational hypertension (or 'pregnancy-induced hypertension') is new hypertension >140/90 mmHg in pregnancy without significant proteinuria.
   b. Pre-eclampsia is a multisystem disorder that usually presents with new-onset hypertension (or new-onset worsening of hypertension) with proteinuria. Pre-eclampsia, particularly in the early stages, may present without proteinuria, but it remains a completely different disease process to gestational hypertension.
   c. Chronic hypertension refers to those women who were hypertensive prior to pregnancy and therefore also at the booking appointment.

2. What are the key points in the history of a woman who presents with raised blood pressure?

   First check for symptoms of pre-eclampsia, which include: severe headache (especially frontal), visual disturbances including blurring and flashing before eyes, severe epigastric/below rib pain, vomiting, sudden oedema of face/hands/feet.

   Then, check for presence of risk factors for pre-eclampsia. High-risk factors include: hypertensive disease during a previous pregnancy, chronic kidney disease, type 1 or type 2 diabetes, chronic hypertension and autoimmune disease such as SLE or antiphospholipid syndrome.

   Moderate risk factors include: first pregnancy, age ≥40 years, pregnancy interval >10 years, raised BMI (≥35 kg/m^2), family history of pre-eclampsia and multiple pregnancy.

3. What investigations would you perform after taking a history and examining the patient?

   Bedside urine dip should be performed to confirm the diagnosis and, if protein ≥1+, a spot protein:creatinine ratio (PCR) or 24-hour urine collection should be used to quantify proteinuria. Significant proteinuria is classified as >30 mg/mmol on PCR or >300 mg protein on 24-hour urine collection.

   Blood tests should be performed to check for complications and include: FBC, clotting, group and save, U&Es, LFTs, uric acid and lactate dehydrogenase (LDH). Classic findings include: low platelets, raised Hb (haemoconcentration) or low Hb (haemolysis), prolonged prothrombin time (PT) and activated partial thromboplastin time (APTT), raised uric acid, LDH, urea, creatinine, transaminases and bilirubin.

Finally, fetal monitoring includes ultrasound for fetal growth and amniotic fluid volume, umbilical artery Doppler velocimetry (if indicated) and CTG.

4. What is the management of diagnosed pre-eclampsia in the absence of severe hypertension or complications?

If pre-eclampsia is diagnosed, the patient should be admitted to hospital for regular BP monitoring (at least four times per day) and monitoring of bloods (at least three times per week). Target BP is <150/80–100 mmHg, and NICE recommends first-line treatment with labetalol. Second-line treatments include methyldopa and nifedipine, though some units use methyldopa as their first-line treatment.

In the absence of complications requiring immediate delivery, the timing of delivery should be decided by a consultant obstetrician, balancing the severity of disease and risk of maternal and fetal complications against fetal maturity. NICE guidance advises the consultant to document a plan for antenatal fetal monitoring and maternal and fetal indications for elective birth before 34 weeks and to deliver at term in cases of mild or moderate hypertension (BP ≤159/109) without any complications.

5. What are the possible complications of pre-eclampsia?

The main fetal complication is IUGR, and there are six maternal complications of pre-eclampsia.

Eclampsia is the development of one or more tonic–clonic convulsions associated with pre-eclampsia and represents severe disease requiring immediate delivery. A warning sign on examination is hyperreflexia and/or clonus ≥3 beats. Treatment is with magnesium sulphate, with a loading dose of 4 g IV over 5 minutes followed by an infusion of 1 g/hour for 24 hours and a further bolus of 2–4 g over 5 minutes if there are recurrent seizures. Magnesium toxicity should be monitored every hour by checking the patellar reflex.

'HELLP' syndrome consists of Haemolysis, Elevated Liver enzymes and Low Platelets and may proceed to disseminated intravascular coagulation. It may present with epigastric/right upper quadrant pain due to liver capsular pain, nausea and vomiting or dark urine due to haemolysis. It also represents severe disease and requires immediate delivery with supportive treatment in the interim and consideration of MgSO$_4$ prophylaxis against eclampsia.

Placental abruption, cerebrovascular haemorrhage due to failure of cerebral autoregulation in severe hypertension, renal failure and pulmonary oedema due to fluid overload or adult respiratory distress syndrome are the four other major complications associated with pre-eclampsia. Good blood pressure control and careful fluid balance are key to prevention.

Complications may develop postnatally, particularly within the first 24 hours, so careful postpartum monitoring is essential.

OBSTETRIC/ANTENATAL EXAMINATION

Score Sheet

Scores: 1 = Not attempted; 2 = Attempted, unsatisfactory; 3 = Attempted, satisfactory

Action	1	2	3
1. **W**ashes hands, **i**ntroduces self to patient, checks patient **i**dentity, explains procedure to patient and obtains **p**ermission, **p**ositions and **e**xposes patient appropriately (WIIPPE)			
2. Takes a brief history of fetal movements from the patient and checks whether the patient is in any pain or discomfort			
3. Performs a general inspection of the patient from the end of the bed and comments on positive and negative findings including skin changes, scars and symmetry			
4. Palpates the abdomen and comments on uterine size and contractions, liquor volume, fetal number and movements, presentation, lie and engagement and measures the symphysis-fundal height (SFH)			
5. Auscultates the abdomen using a Pinard's stethoscope or listens to the heartbeat using a Sonicaid and comments on the rate			
6. Offers to check the patient for signs of pre-eclampsia, gestational diabetes, anaemia and infection			
7. Thanks the patient, allows her to dress in privacy, then presents findings to examiner			
Overall score		/21	

1. All clinical examinations should begin with these simple checks. It is important to explain to the patient exactly what you are going to do, particularly with regard to palpation, and you should always offer a chaperone. The appropriate exposure is from xiphisternum to pubic symphysis, and the ideal position is lying flat on the couch as for an abdominal exam, usually with a pillow to raise the head slightly for comfort.

2. Before starting the antenatal examination, in addition to checking whether the patient is in or has been experiencing any pain, it is important to check whether she has felt any fetal movements and, if so, what gestation they first started, their frequency and whether there has been any recent change. It is normal to first feel fetal movements between weeks 16 and 25 and for them to become well established by week 28. After 28 weeks, baby movements should be felt at least 10 times over a 2-hour period.

3. From the end of the bed, look particularly for:
   a. **Skin changes**
      i. Linea nigra: a central, dark, pigmented line extending upwards from the symphysis pubis
      ii. Striae gravidarum: purple/red depressed streaks (stretch marks) extending downwards across the abdomen from the current gestation

iii. Striae albicans: striae gravidarum turn silver/white after delivery and, so, their presence indicates previous gestation(s)

These skin changes are normal in pregnancy.

b. **Scars**

i. Pfannenstiel scar from previous 'lower section' caesarean section (transverse incision just above the bikini line)

ii. Laparotomy scar from previous abdominal surgery/'classical' caesarean section (vertical incision in the midline)

iii. Laparoscopy scars from previous keyhole surgery (small 5–10 mm port site scars, below the umbilicus and in any quadrant of the abdomen)

c. **Symmetry:** Asymmetry of abdominal distension can provide clues to fetal number, lie and presentation prior to palpation

4. Ask once again about any pain in the abdomen before beginning palpation. Then, using both hands, assess for:

a. **Uterine size:** The uterus is just palpable at 12 weeks, is in line with the umbilicus at 20 weeks and is at the level of the xiphisternum at 36 weeks.

b. **Contractions:** Strength, duration, location and whether the mother feels them.

c. **Liquor volume:** If the fetal parts are difficult to palpate, it may indicate excessive liquor volume (polyhydramnios). This can be idiopathic but may also indicate underlying pathology such as gestational diabetes or congenital abnormalities. If the fetal parts are very easy to palpate, it may indicate reduced liquor volume (oligohydramnios). This may indicate an underlying abnormality with the fetus' renal tract or premature rupture of the membranes.

d. **Fetal number:** A large uterus may indicate a multiple pregnancy, and this can be confirmed by palpation of two fetal heads and auscultation of two fetal heartbeats (>10 bpm variance).

e. **Movements:** During the course of palpation, it is normally possible to appreciate fetal movements; however, if the fetus is sleeping and is not awoken by the examination, then you may not feel any.

f. **Presentation:** The presentation of the fetus is the part that 'presents' at the pelvic inlet, and can be cephalic (head) or breech (buttock). There are various ways of assessing presentation; one method is to use the thumb and index finger of one hand to press firmly just above the pubic symphysis. This will allow you to distinguish between cephalic presentation (head in pelvic inlet, therefore a hard, round shape palpable) and breech presentation (buttock in pelvic inlet, therefore a soft, broad shape palpable). You can then palpate the opposite end to corroborate your findings, though bear in mind that even in the most experienced hands, it can sometimes be difficult to tell! Note also that the pelvic inlet may feel empty if the lie is transverse.

g. **Lie:** The lie of the fetus relates to the position of the fetus' back:
  i. **Longitudinal lie** indicates that the back is lying longitudinally, from pubic symphysis to xiphisternum (breech or cephalic).
  ii. **Transverse lie** indicates that the back is lying transversely, from flank to flank (head and buttocks palpable in the flanks as opposed to the pelvic inlet).
  iii. **Oblique lie** indicates that the back is lying obliquely, from left iliac fossa to right upper quadrant or right iliac fossa to left upper quadrant (head and buttocks palpable in opposite quadrants as opposed to the pelvic inlet).
h. **Engagement:** The engagement of the fetus relates to how much of the fetal head has entered the pelvic brim. It is measured as the number of finger breadths or 'fifths' of head that are palpable at the pelvic inlet (because the part of the head that has entered the true pelvis is no longer palpable). When 50% of the head (and therefore the widest part) has entered, it is said to be 'engaged'. Accordingly, when the fetal head is palpable by two fingers (two-fifths) or less, it is said to be engaged; when it is palpable by three fingers (three-fifths) or more, it is said to be not engaged.

Engagement is the first of the seven stages or 'cardinal movements' of normal labour:

Stage	Description
Engagement	Fetal head enters pelvic inlet, as the biparietal diameter (ear to ear) descends into the pelvic inlet and the occiput is at the level of the ischial spines
Descent	Downward movement of the head through the pelvis with contractions
Flexion	Flexion of the baby's head with the chin meeting the chest, allowing the smallest diameter of the baby's head to present into the pelvis
Internal rotation	Rotation of the baby in line with the change in shape of the pelvis from inlet (widest left to right) to outlet (widest front to back) so that the baby directly faces the mother's spine
Extension	Extension of the baby's head to deliver the top of the head, face and chin
External rotation/ restitution	Rotation of the baby from facing the mother's spine to facing left or right, in order to allow delivery of the shoulders
Expulsion	Delivery of the anterior shoulder, then the posterior shoulder and then the rest of the baby's body with an upward motion

i. **SFH:** Establish the position of the fundus of the uterus by pressing down with the ulnar border of the hand, starting at the xiphisternum and moving inferiorly, until firm resistance is felt. Use a tape measure to measure from this point to the pubic symphysis, normally using the unmarked side to avoid bias, and then turn the tape around to reveal the SFH. From 20 to 36 weeks, the SFH approximates to the gestation of the pregnancy within ±2 weeks, as it increases by 1 cm/week.

5. Some OSCE examiners will require you to be able to use a Pinard's stethoscope, though in clinical practice a Sonicaid (Doppler fetal monitor) is almost always used, and so this may be all that is required. With either method, first locate the anterior shoulder of the fetus based upon your assessment of presentation and lie because this will be where the fetal heart is best heard (for a cephalic presentation, this will be in the left or right lower quadrant, and for breech presentation, this will be in the left or right upper quadrant).

   For the Pinard's stethoscope method, position it over where you think the anterior shoulder is, place your ear against it and then remove your hands. For the Sonicaid method, place some ultrasound gel on the probe and place it in the same position. Comment on the fetal heartbeat, which should be between 110 and 160 bpm. If you are unsure whether you are listening to the mother's heartbeat, you can palpate the radial pulse at the same time or auscultate the heart to ascertain maternal heart rate.

6. To complete the examination, you should offer to examine the patient and perform simple bedside tests for pre-eclampsia, gestational diabetes, anaemia and infection.
   a. Offer to examine for peripheral and central oedema (pre-eclampsia) and for conjunctival pallor (anaemia)
   b. Offer to check the mother's temperature (infection), heart rate and respiratory rate for tachycardia and tachypnoea (anaemia) and blood pressure for hypertension (pre-eclampsia)
   c. Offer to check the urine for leucocytes and nitrites (infection), proteinuria (pre-eclampsia) and glucose (gestational diabetes)

7. Thank the patient and allow her to dress in privacy, and then present your findings to the examiner. An example presentation for a normal antenatal examination would be:

> *I was asked to perform an antenatal examination on Mrs P, a 26-year-old woman who presented for a routine antenatal check at 36 weeks for her first pregnancy. The patient has felt the baby move around 10 times an hour, as has been normal over the last month and has not experienced any abdominal pain. On inspection there is a linea nigra visible as a pigmented line in the midline and purple longitudinal streaks consistent with striae gravidarum visible on either side. There are no previous scars suggestive of caesarean sections or abdominal surgery. On palpation, the fundus of the uterus is palpable at the xiphisternum indicating a 36-week pregnancy and there are no contractions. There is only one fetus palpable, and the ease of palpation of the fetal parts is suggestive of normal liquor volume. The presentation is cephalic, the lie is longitudinal, and the*

head is *five-fifths palpable and is not engaged. The SFH is 36 cm, and the fetal heart rate as measured with a Sonicaid is 140–150 bpm.*

In summary, this is a normal antenatal examination of a 26-year-old woman who is 36 weeks' pregnant in her first gestation. The fetus is growing as expected, with normal liquor volume and healthy heart rate, and is presently cephalic.

I would complete the examination by assessing the patient for central and peripheral oedema suggestive of pre-eclampsia and conjunctival pallor suggestive of anaemia; take the patient's blood pressure to assess for pre-eclampsia; and take a urine dip to check for glucose (in gestational diabetes), protein (in pre-eclampsia) and leucocytes and nitrites (in urinary tract infections).

2: Paediatrics

GENERAL PAEDIATRIC HISTORY

History taking involves utilizing communication skills to gather information in a structured process and, so, marks will be allocated for: (1) communication skills, (2) structure and (3) the completeness of the information that you obtain. From the outset, you should keep in mind that a good history does not involve blindly asking the same list of questions and presenting your findings. Instead, it involves developing an initial differential diagnosis of the most likely causes for the symptoms based upon the presenting complaints and employing a thoughtful and logical approach to narrowing this down through relevant questions to formulate a diagnosis and a management plan. This approach will not only score you high marks in the exam but will serve to help you manage patients better in clinical practice.

Score Sheet

Scores: 1 = Not attempted; 2 = Attempted, unsatisfactory; 3 = Attempted, satisfactory

Action	1	2	3
1. Introduces self to child and accompanying adult appropriately and develops rapport suitable for the child's age			
2. Elicits the child's presenting complaints			
3. Elicits the history of each presenting complaint and any associated symptoms			
4. Establishes the impact of the illness on the child and the family and identifies any ideas or concerns the carer has about the illness			
5. Obtains a complete past medical history, including medical conditions, previous surgery, GP and hospital presentations and admissions			
6. Obtains a pregnancy and birth history, including antenatal, intrapartum and neonatal issues			
7. Obtains a relevant feeding and dietary history			
8. Obtains a relevant growth and developmental history			
9. Obtains a drug and allergy history			
10. Obtains a complete immunization history			
11. Obtains a complete family history and constructs an appropriate pedigree chart			

Continued

Action	1	2	3
12. Obtains an appropriate social history, taking into account home and school settings and any recent travel			
13. Checks main details with the patient/parent			
14. Presents the history and summarizes key findings			
Overall score		/42	

1. An important principle in paediatric history taking is adapting your approach to the age of the child, particularly with respect to your vocabulary. If the patient is an infant, this will simply involve making sure the patient is engaged for the duration of the history. With younger children, you should introduce yourself to them before introducing yourself to the carer and make sure that there are age-appropriate toys to keep them engaged. With older children, it is good practice to focus the history taking on them, referring to the carer only after the child has fully answered each question. In some cases, for example if the carer keeps intervening during a consultation with a teenager, it may be more appropriate to take the history with the patient and the carer separately (if the patient consents).

   A good general approach to opening a paediatric history station is to first introduce yourself to the child and carer, then to establish the relationship of the child to the carer and to any others present in the room. During the initial introduction, you should check the full name and date of birth of the child to ensure you are seeing the correct patient and clarify the referral source (brought in by ambulance, walked-in, referred by GP).

   It is also important to establish a friendly atmosphere to make sure the child is comfortable, which can involve smiling, providing toys, positioning the child on the carer's lap or, in the case of a teenager, just addressing the patient directly and developing rapport.

2. The presenting complaint should be elicited from the child or carer as appropriate with an open question, for example, 'What's brought you in to see us today?' Patients may have more than one presenting complaint, for example diarrhoea and vomiting, or fever and cough, in which case you should document each symptom in the patient's own words and take a history of presenting complaint for each.

3. For each symptom, a history of presenting complaint should be obtained. You should always start by asking when the child was last completely well, so as not to miss the early symptoms. Common examples include:

Presenting complaint	History of presenting complaint
Pain	Use the 'SOCRATES' tool: **Site:** Where is the pain now and does that differ from where it was when it first started?

Continued

Presenting complaint	History of presenting complaint
	Onset: Is the pain acute or chronic; when did it start; did it come on suddenly, over a minute or so or more gradually? What was the child doing at the time of onset and were there any unwell contacts? **Character:** What is the nature of the pain (sharp, dull, burning or gripping)? Try not to put words into the patient's mouth, instead document their answer in their own words. **Radiation:** Does the pain spread to anywhere else or is it fixed in that spot? **Associated symptoms:** For chest pain, ask about shortness of breath, cough, wheeze, palpitations, sweating, nausea and vomiting; for abdominal pain, ask about diarrhoea, blood in stools, constipation, bloating, nausea and vomiting; for pain elsewhere, ask about any other appropriate symptoms. **Timing:** Is the pain constant or intermittent; what is the frequency; are there precipitating factors or is it always there; is it getting better or worse; any past history of a similar pain? **Exacerbating and relieving factors:** Does anything make the pain better or worse; for example, is it better lying still or moving around; is it better if they take shallow breaths; is it worse after exercise? Have they tried using simple analgesia such as Calpol (paracetamol) and Neurofen (ibuprofen)? **Severity:** For example, on a scale of 1–10, how bad is the pain? Or use a validated pain scoring tool depending on the age of the child.
Cough	**Onset and timing:** When did it start; is it constant or worse during the day or night; are there any precipitating factors or is it always there; is it getting better or worse; any unwell contacts; any past history of cough? **Character:** What does the cough sound like (wet, dry, barking, whooping)? Again, document the patient's or carer's description instead of putting words in their mouth: is it productive, and if so, what colour is the sputum? **Associated symptoms:** Is there any wheeze, fever, shortness of breath or chest pain? Any history of eczema, hay fever, allergies or family history of asthma or atopy? **Exacerbating and relieving factors:** Does anything make the cough better or worse; for example, is it worse on exercise, on being outside, at night?
Fever	**Onset and timing:** When did the fever start; is it constant or does it come and go; any recent travel abroad, any unwell contacts? **Associated symptoms:** Any lethargy, drowsiness or reduced appetite; any rashes; any rigors/shaking or fits; any signs of meningism (headache, neck stiffness or photophobia); any night sweats; any respiratory, gastrointestinal or genitourinary symptoms (see Systems review below for full details)? **Exacerbating and relieving factors:** Any improvement with analgesia?
Rash	**Site:** Where is the rash now and does that differ from when it was first noticed; has it spread and what is the pattern? **Onset and timing:** When did the patient first notice the rash; could anything have precipitated the rash; any travel or unwell contacts; is the rash spreading or getting better; any history of a similar rash? **Character:** What does the rash look like; what colour is it; does it blanch; does it itch?

Continued

Presenting complaint	History of presenting complaint
	Associated symptoms: Any lethargy, drowsiness or reduced appetite; any documented fever, meningism (see above), respiratory or gastrointestinal symptoms?
Diarrhoea	**Onset and timing:** When did the diarrhoea start; how frequent are the motions; could anything have precipitated the diarrhoea; any travel or unwell contacts; is it getting better or worse; any previous history of diarrhoea?
	Character: Is the stool watery, loose or well-formed but frequent; is there any blood or mucus?
	Associated symptoms: Any abdominal pain and is it associated with feeding, any nausea or vomiting, fever or urinary symptoms (dysuria, frequency/ oliguria, urgency/enuresis, hesitancy/poor stream)?
Vomiting	**Onset and timing:** When did the vomiting start; how many times and how frequently is the patient vomiting; could anything be precipitating the vomiting; is it related to food, any travel or unwell contacts; any previous history of vomiting?
	Character: What is the colour and content of the vomit; is it food or bilious; is there any blood; is it projectile?
	Associated symptoms: Any abdominal pain, nausea, diarrhoea, fever or urinary symptoms?
Seizures, fits or funny turns	Use the background before, during and after approach to structure a history of presenting complaint for a seizure and tailor the questions to the age of the child.
	Background: Any fever (febrile convulsions are the most common cause of fits in younger children) or has the child been unwell recently; any history or family history of epilepsy, heart disease, migraine, fainting episodes, hyperventilation, breath-holding or developmental concerns; any trauma or emotional/unpleasant events preceding the seizure?
	Before: Any prodrome or aura; how long did this last?
	During: How long did it last; any loss of consciousness; any movement or jerking of limbs and what was the pattern (did it start on one side and then become generalized or was it generalized from the onset?); any tongue biting or urinary/faecal incontinence; did they injure themselves at all?
	After: Any drowsiness or confusion; any memory of the event; any residual neurology; how long did it take for them to get back to their normal self?
Headache	**Site:** What is the site of the headache; is it frontal, on one side, occipital, behind the eyes or more of a facial pain; has that changed since?
	Onset: Is it acute or chronic; when did it start; did it come on suddenly, over a minute or so, or more gradually; was there any aura; what was the child doing at the time; any unwell contacts?
	Character: What is the nature of the headache (sharp, dull, tight band, throbbing)?
	Associated symptoms: Any fever or signs of meningism; any nausea or vomiting, visual symptoms (flickering of light, blurred vision), weakness, seizures, change in behaviour or deterioration in school performance?
	Timing: Is it constant or intermittent; what is the frequency and is this changing; are there any precipitating factors, e.g. food, stress, light, noise; is it worse in the morning or does it wake them at night; is it/are they getting better or worse?

Continued

Presenting complaint	History of presenting complaint
	Exacerbating and relieving factors: Does anything make the headaches better or worse, e.g. bright lights, lying down, taking simple analgesia? **Severity:** For example, a pain score of 1–10 or use a validated pain scoring tool for younger children. In the **past medical history** ask about any ventriculoperitoneal (VP)/ ventriculoatrial (VA) shunts, any recent illnesses including visual problems, dental problems, earache or sinusitis, and in the **family history** ask about migraines.
Systems review	**Neurological:** Headache, head injury, fainting or dizziness, funny fits or turns, weakness, numbness, clumsiness or abnormal gait. Any change in school performance or loss of skills? **Ophthalmological:** Red eyes, discharge, change in vision, double vision or squint. **Upper respiratory tract/ear, nose and throat:** Ear pain, difficulty hearing, discharge from ear canal, surgery or grommets, runny nose, nosebleeds, sore throat, difficulty swallowing, neck lumps or stiffness. **Lower respiratory tract/chest:** Chest pain, shortness of breath, wheeze, stridor, cough, sputum, cyanosis. **Cardiovascular:** Chest pain, palpitations, sweating, sudden collapse, poor feeding, failure to thrive/gain weight. **Gastrointestinal:** Abdominal pain or distension, diarrhoea, constipation, vomiting, jaundice, reduced appetite, bloody stools. **Genitourinary:** Dysuria, frequency, oliguria, urgency, enuresis, hesitancy, poor stream, haematuria, urethral or vaginal discharge or itching. **Musculoskeletal:** Joint or limb pain, swelling or deformity, difficulty walking or moving limbs. **Dermatological:** Rashes, eczema or dry skin, itching, hives or easy bruising/ bleeding.

4. Having taken the history of each presenting complaint, it is also important to establish how the symptoms are affecting the child's life and the family's life. An example may be a nocturnal cough that has resulted in the child not being able to sleep and being tired and unable to concentrate in school, with the parent also being kept up at night and being less productive at work. These questions are important because they provide a context to the illness and allow you to tailor your management plan to address the needs of the child and the family.

In a similar vein, it is important to establish any ideas that the carer may have about the cause of the symptoms and any concerns that the carer may have. This should be elicited with direct questions; for example, 'Do you have any ideas as to what may be causing John's cough?' and 'Do you have any particular concerns or worries about John's cough?' By addressing the carer's concerns directly and developing his or her understanding, the carer will be more engaged in the 'shared' management plan, which will increase compliance. It may also uncover any unarticulated fears or hidden agendas, which can then be addressed. Some people prefer to leave this line of questioning until the end of the history taking; it is just a matter of personal preference.

5. The past medical history should include:
   a. **Any medical conditions** (e.g. eczema, asthma, epilepsy, diabetes) or previous illnesses and whether these are ongoing/active or resolved/inactive.
   b. **Previous presentations** to GP or A&E, outpatient appointments and hospital admissions with duration of stay and management.
   c. **Surgical history**, with date, operation and complications.

6. The pregnancy and birth history should include:
   a. **Antenatal:** Health of the mother in pregnancy, any diabetes or raised blood pressure, any antenatal infections, any abnormalities on antenatal blood tests or ultrasound scans, such as intrauterine growth retardation, and medications taken during pregnancy that may be teratogenic?
   b. **Intrapartum:** Gestation, mode of delivery (normal vaginal delivery, forceps, ventouse or caesarean section), birthweight, condition of the baby at delivery (e.g. APGAR score if the parents know it).
   c. **Neonatal:** Any immediate issues at birth/SCBU admissions, any health problems in the first weeks of life, particularly with feeding?

7. The feeding and dietary history is important for two reasons: first, if a child is off their feeds, it may be an indicator of the severity of the illness, possibly requiring admission for fluid resuscitation. Second, a dietary factor may be responsible for the symptom complex, for example, an allergy or gluten in the presentation of coeliac disease. Like all sections, this should also be adapted to the age of the child:
   a. **Infants:** Are/were they breast fed or formula fed; what type of formula; how much with each feed; how often are they fed; what age were they weaned onto solids and were there any problems with weaning; what is the range of foods eaten? Always ask about intake in the last 24 hours and whether this is different from the average intake.
   b. **Toddlers and older children:** Were they breast fed or formula fed; what is their typical diet now and has it changed recently (particularly if the child is presenting with gastrointestinal symptoms)?

8. Ask the carer whether he or she has any concerns about the child's height or weight and, if appropriate, review the child's red book and record height, weight and head circumference on the growth centile charts.

   Ask whether there are any developmental concerns, which, for an infant or toddler, would include questions on developmental milestones with regard to gross motor skills, fine motor skills, language, social development and concerns about hearing and vision. For an older child, questions about development would be more related to performance at school and whether there have been any changes or deterioration.

9. The drug history includes the child's current medications, dosage, frequency, date started and any changes in regime since the start date. It is

also worth asking who commenced the medication (GP or paediatrician) and enquiring into any old medications that have since been stopped. As is usual, it is also important to take an allergy history, to drugs, foodstuffs (e.g. nuts, shellfish, egg, gluten) and contact allergies.

10. It is important to check whether the child's immunizations are up to date and, if not, why not. This is another area where it is important to explore the parent's reasons for omitting any immunizations and to counsel them appropriately. If the parent is unsure, you can check in the red book if he or she has it with him or her or with the child's GP. Some people prefer to ask about the drug and immunization history after the past medical history; again, it is a matter of personal preference.

11. An important aspect of establishing whether there are any illnesses that run in the family is drawing a pedigree chart. This should include siblings, parents and grandparents and, if there is a positive family history of genetic disease, all known affected relatives. Once you have drawn a pedigree chart with the ages of each individual, you can then detail any medical conditions or whether anybody is acutely unwell, age and cause of death and consanguinity. Consanguinity can be an awkward thing to establish, but a direct question is the best way to approach it, such as 'Are you and your partner related by blood?'

   Pedigree charts are discussed in the Data Interpretation section.

12. The social history can be split into life at home and at school:
    a. **Home:** Who lives at home, any regular visitors (e.g. carers), occupation of any adults in the house, any problems at home, any smokers, any pets, any recent travel abroad, any unwell contacts, any changes in mood or behaviour, any changes in sleep patterns?
    b. **School:** How is the child doing at school, any recent changes in schoolwork, school friends or any bullying?

13. Paediatric histories can contain a lot of information, and it can be helpful to clarify the key points, particularly in relation to the history of each presenting complaint and to any other positive findings in the history. This will also allow you to order your thoughts before presenting your findings to the examiner.

14. An example for a typical presentation of acute otitis media would be:

John is a 3-year-old boy who has been brought in by his mum with a 3-day history of right ear pain and a 1-day history of fever up to 38.5°C. There has been no discharge, itchiness or loss of hearing from the ear, no history of swimming, and the fever has been well controlled with regular Calpol. He has no respiratory or urinary symptoms, no diarrhoea or vomiting and is off his food but still drinking well. He is otherwise fit and well with no medical conditions and has only visited his GP for mild viral illnesses that have self-resolved. He was born at term by normal vaginal delivery after an uneventful pregnancy, weighing 3.5 kg, and was discharged home the same day. He had no issues in the neonatal period. He normally feeds well and eats a good range of family foods and is growing well, and there are no developmental concerns. He is not on any medications other than Calpol for the fever and has no allergies, and immunizations are up to date. He lives at home with mum, dad and older sister Kate, all of whom are fit and well. There are no smokers at home, no pets and no history of recent travel, though John attends a nursery where several of the children have had coughs and colds recently. Mum is concerned because one of the children became very unwell and needed antibiotics before they became better.

In summary, this is a 3-year-old boy who is normally fit and well, presenting with a history of right ear pain and fever consistent with a diagnosis of acute otitis media.

CLINICAL SCENARIO: WHEEZE

Wheeze is a common presentation in childhood, with age being a good indicator towards the most common causes: bronchiolitis in babies under 9 months and asthma in older children. Viral-induced wheeze is a diagnosis applied to young children who present with a wheeze with an upper respiratory tract infection. It can progress to asthma but does not always do so. Inhaled foreign body and heart failure are two important differential diagnoses that must not be missed.

Typical findings in the history for each diagnosis include:

Diagnosis	Features on history
Bronchiolitis	Most cases under 9 months of age
	Winter epidemics
	Cough, coryza and respiratory distress that may progress to apnoeas
	Poor feeding
Viral-induced wheeze	Most cases between 6 months and 5 years of age
	Symptoms of an upper respiratory tract infection, e.g. cough, coryza, fever
	Past history of bronchiolitis may be present
	No history of wheeze in the absence of infection
Asthma	Recurrent episodes of cough and wheeze in the absence of infection
	Nocturnal cough is often present and may be the only symptom
	Past history or family history of atopy (asthma, eczema, hay fever, allergies)
	Triggers, e.g. pollen, smoke, dust, pets, cold, infections and exercise
Heart failure	Poor feeding, respiratory distress and failure to thrive
	Most clues are on examination: crackles, murmur, displaced apex and hepatomegaly
Inhaled foreign body	Most cases in toddlers
	History of playing with toys or small objects then choking
	Sudden onset wheeze, normally systemically well
	May have stridor if the obstruction is high

Case 1: asthma
Presentation

Jamie is a 6-year-old boy who has been brought in by his mum having developed wheeze, chest tightness and difficulty breathing while *running at school, with a respiratory rate of 30, a heart rate of 100 and a temperature of 36.8°C. This has happened a few times over the last year while doing sport, but it is worse today than it has been previously. He is otherwise fit and well with no medical conditions, though he did suffer from eczema as a child. He was born at term by normal vaginal delivery after an uneventful pregnancy, weighing 3.8 kg, and was discharged home the same day. He had no issues in the neonatal period. He has a good diet and is growing well, and there are no developmental concerns. He is not on any medications and suffers from mild hay fever, and immunizations are up to date. He lives at home with mum and dad, and his mother had asthma as a child. The house is well ventilated, and there are no smokers at home, no pets and no history of recent travel. Mum is concerned because he loves sport, and she is worried that he will have to stop.*

In summary, this is a 6-year-old boy with a past history of eczema and hay fever and a mother who had asthma as a child, presenting with exercise-induced wheeze on a background of similar but less severe presentations. These findings are consistent with a diagnosis of acute asthma.

Other possible findings

1. Current: nocturnal cough, trigger-induced wheeze including smokers at home.
2. Past medical history: viral-induced wheeze as a younger child, preterm delivery, smoking during pregnancy, premature delivery.

Questions

(Answers based on current Scottish Intercollegiate Guidelines Network (SIGN)/British Thoracic Society (BTS) guidelines)

1. The underlying cause of asthma is unknown, but there are known risk factors – what are they?
   Possible risk factors for asthma include: personal or family history of asthma or atopy (eczema, hay fever, rhinitis, allergies), prematurity/low birthweight and maternal or personal history of smoking; past history of bronchiolitis and viral-induced wheeze. More recent evidence also suggests that childhood obesity increases the risk and severity of asthma.

2. What are some of the features on history and examination that would lower the likelihood of a diagnosis of asthma?
   Clinical features that lower the probability of asthma include: symptoms appearing only with viral infections with no interval symptoms, moist cough, normal chest examination, spirometry or peak expiratory flow (PEF) while symptomatic, no response to a trial of bronchodilators. Clinical features pointing to an alternative diagnosis, e.g. foreign body or heart failure, would also lower the probability of an asthma diagnosis.

3. What is the role of spirometry in the diagnosis of asthma in children?

Based on the history and examination, a child can be classed into one of three groups:

High probability – diagnosis of asthma likely

Intermediate probability – diagnosis uncertain

Low probability – diagnosis other than asthma likely

In children with an intermediate probability of asthma who are old enough to perform spirometry (most children over 5), it can be used to support the diagnosis as likely or unlikely. If there is evidence of airways obstruction (i.e. while the child is symptomatic), the change in forced expiratory volume in one second (FEV_1) or peak expiratory flow (PEF) should be assessed in response to an inhaled bronchodilator. If there is significant reversibility, which is the hallmark of asthma, then a diagnosis of asthma is probable and a trial of treatment should be commenced. If there is no significant reversibility, then a diagnosis other than asthma is likely and the child should be referred for further testing.

An alternative approach for children with an intermediate probability of asthma, particularly for children too young to perform spirometry, is to proceed as with high probability and commence a trial of treatment, review and assess response.

4. What is the stepwise approach to the treatment of asthma in children?

The stepwise approach involves starting treatment of asthma at the step most appropriate to the initial severity to achieve early control, then maintaining control by stepping up treatment as necessary and stepping back down when treatment is good. Stepping up should always be preceded by checking inhaler technique, compliance and possible elimination of trigger factors.

In children aged 5–12 years, the stepwise approach is:

a. Step 1 (mild intermittent asthma)
   i. Inhaled short-acting β_2 agonist as required
b. Step 2 (regular preventer therapy)
   i. Add inhaled steroid 200–400 µg/day
c. Step 3 (initial add-on therapy)
   i. Add inhaled long-acting β_2 agonist (LABA)
   ii. Assess control
   iii. If good response to LABA, continue
   iv. If benefit but control inadequate, increase inhaled steroid dose to 400 µg/day
   v. If no response, stop LABA and increase inhaled steroid dose to 400 µg/day
   vi. If control still inadequate, start trial of leukotriene receptor antagonist or sustained-release theophylline
d. Step 4 (persistent poor control)
   i. Increase inhaled steroid dose up to 800 µg/day

e. Step 5 (oral steroids)
   i. Use daily steroid tablet in lowest dose to provide adequate control, while maintaining inhaled steroids at 800 μg/day
   ii. Refer to respiratory paediatrician if not already done

5. What are the features of acute severe and life-threatening asthma?
   The features of acute severe asthma in children include: SpO$_2$ <92%, PEF 33%–50% best/predicted, HR >125/min and RR >30/min (>5 years) or HR >140/min and RR >40/min (2–5 years) and cannot complete sentences in one breath or too breathless to talk or feed.

   The features of life-threatening asthma in children include: PEF <33% best/predicted, hypotension, poor respiratory effort, silent chest, cyanosis, exhaustion, confusion and coma.

6. What is the distinction between viral-induced wheeze and asthma?
   Viral-induced wheeze is a distinct diagnosis from asthma, with a different underlying mechanism and variable response to bronchodilators. It only occurs with an infection, e.g. upper respiratory tract infection, with no interval symptoms and generally only between 6 months and 5 years of age. It is important to make the distinction because there is little evidence to suggest a trial of treatment in these children, and it can be difficult to distinguish the response to treatment and spontaneous improvement due to resolution of the viral infection. It is, however, reasonable to prescribe a short-acting bronchodilator and montelukast to be used as soon as the child becomes symptomatic in future episodes in these children if they show a good response to treatment.

Case 2: bronchiolitis

Presentation

Louise is a 6-month-old girl who has been brought in by her mum in with rapid breathing and wheeze, a SpO$_2$ of 94% and poor feeding, on a background of a cough and runny nose for the last 2 days. She is otherwise fit and well with no medical conditions. She was born at term by normal vaginal delivery after an uneventful pregnancy, weighing 3.2 kg, and was discharged home the same day. She had no issues in the neonatal period. She is still breastfeeding well and is growing above the twenty-fifth centile, and there are no developmental concerns. She is not on any medications and has no allergies, and immunizations are up to date. She lives at home with mum and dad, and there is no significant family history. There are no smokers at home, no pets and no history of recent travel. Mum is really worried as this is her first child and she was not sure if this was a normal cold or something more serious.

In summary, this is a 6-month-old girl with difficulty breathing and poor feeding on the background of a coryzal illness and no other significant history. These findings are consistent with a diagnosis of bronchiolitis.

Other possible findings

1. Current: apnoeas, other signs of respiratory distress including tachycardia, hyperinflation, intercostal and subcostal recession, tracheal tug and cyanosis.
2. Past medical history: prematurity, chronic lung disease, congenital heart disease.

Questions

1. What are the causative organisms for bronchiolitis?

   The main causative organism for bronchiolitis is respiratory syncytial virus, which accounts for around 80% of cases. The other causative organisms are all viruses, including adenovirus, influenza and parainfluenza.

2. What are the indications for admission in cases of bronchiolitis?

   Indications for admission include low oxygen saturations, signs of respiratory distress or apnoeas, poor feeding or, as in this case, parental anxiety.

3. What is the most serious complication of bronchiolitis?

   The most serious complication is bronchiolitis obliterans. This rare complication occurs most commonly with adenovirus bronchiolitis and causes permanent damage to the small airways. The more common complication to warn parents about is the development of viral-induced wheeze in the early years following bronchiolitis.

CLINICAL SCENARIO: THE FITTING CHILD

The fitting child is a common history-taking station in paediatrics as it is a presentation that is very worrying for parents and has a slightly different structure for history taking to other presenting complaints.

The differential is broad and typical findings in the history for common diagnoses include:

Diagnosis	Features on history
Syncope/ vasovagal episode	Before: lightheadedness, closing in of visual fields and pallor, typically occurs when standing up, never while lying down
	During: short period of unresponsiveness, may have jerking/twitching of fine amplitude and/or urinary incontinence
	After: rapid recovery but may feel tired
Febrile convulsion	Before: most aged 6 months to 5 years, high temperature
	During: typical generalized tonic–clonic seizure, lasting less than 15 minutes, may include urinary or faecal incontinence and/or tongue biting
	After: may have short post-ictal phase and feel tired afterwards but with complete neurological recovery
Reflex anoxic seizure	Before: most occur in 1–3 year olds, precipitated by an unpleasant event, e.g. physical or emotional trauma, sudden onset of pallor followed by loss of tone and consciousness

Continued

Diagnosis	Features on history
	During: short period of unresponsiveness, may have tonic or tonic–clonic seizures, upward eye movement and/or urinary incontinence After: rapid recovery but may feel tired
Breath-holding spell	Before: occur in infants and toddlers under the age of 5, typical pattern of an unpleasant event, e.g. physical/emotional trauma leading to crying then holding breath in prolonged expiration, resulting in cyanosis (hence the term 'blue' breath-holding spell) and loss of tone and consciousness During: period of unconsciousness of a few minutes that may be associated with fine amplitude tonic–clonic jerking After: rapid recovery but may feel tired
Tonic–clonic 'grand mal' epileptic seizure	Before: may be precipitated by an aura (which older children will be able to describe better than younger children) or may begin with sudden onset loss of consciousness and falling down, which may be associated with an expiratory grunt During: initial 'tonic' phase of contraction of limbs with eyes rolled back, followed by 'clonic' phase of rhythmic jerking, often associated with urinary and faecal incontinence and/or tongue biting, silent throughout After: post-ictal phase of unconsciousness followed by confusion and drowsiness lasting up to an hour and amnesia related to the event
Pseudoseizure	Before: most common in adolescents, in the presence of others, often on a background (on detailed history taking) of emotional, physical or sexual abuse or difficulties During: variable presentation with bizarre, non-rhythmic movements of the limbs and eyes, without cyanosis, pallor, incontinence or tongue biting, may groan throughout in contrast to true epileptic seizures, which are silent during the tonic–clonic phase After: variable recovery, may be rapid, may express disorientation or amnesia, distinguishable from true post-ictal phase

Case 1: febrile convulsion

Presentation

Avani is a 2-year-old girl who has been brought in by her dad having gone stiff and then jerking her arms and legs rhythmically for around 2 minutes, during which time she passed urine. She could not be roused during the episode and was quite difficult to rouse for the first 15 minutes after the episode on the way to hospital but is alert and responsive now. She has had a runny nose and high fever for 1 day, which the GP has diagnosed as a viral upper respiratory tract infection, but her temperature at home has been up to 38.5°C. She is otherwise fit and well with no medical conditions and has never had a seizure before today. She was born at term by elective caesarean section for breech presentation after an uneventful pregnancy, weighing 3.2 kg, and had no issues in the neonatal period. She is feeding well and is growing along the fiftieth centile, and there are no developmental concerns. She is not on any medications other than Calpol and Neurofen for the fever and has no allergies, and immunizations are up to date. She lives at home with mum and dad and her

5-year-old brother, all of whom are well, and there is no significant family history. There are no smokers at home, no pets and no history of recent travel. Dad is really worried that this might be epilepsy.

In summary, this is a 2-year-old girl who has presented with loss of consciousness, rhythmic jerking of all four limbs lasting 2 minutes and associated urinary incontinence on a background of high fever. These findings are consistent with a diagnosis of febrile convulsion.

Other possible findings
1. Current: faecal incontinence or tongue biting, may last longer.
2. Family history of febrile seizures.

Questions
1. What is a febrile convulsion and what is its relationship to epilepsy?

   A febrile convulsion is a convulsion secondary to a febrile illness in a child, normally aged between 6 months and 5 years. They can be simple (generalized tonic–clonic seizure lasting less than 15 minutes with no recurrence within 24 hours or the same illness) or complex (one or more of: focal features, lasting more than 15 minutes, recurrence within 24 hours or the same illness, or incomplete recovery within 1 hour).

   They are not epileptic seizures, but the risk of developing epilepsy if a child has had a simple febrile convulsion is approximately 2.4% compared with 1.4% in the general population. This risk further increases if the child has had a complex febrile convulsion, there are abnormal neurological signs or there is a family history of epilepsy.

2. What further advice would you give parents about the chance of it happening again and what to do if it does?

   Approximately 30% of children who have a febrile convulsion will have a further febrile convulsion in the future. If this occurs, the advice to be given to parents includes:
   a. Stay calm, and note the time of onset
   b. If they are in a safe position, do not move them, try to stop the jerking or put anything in their mouths
   c. If it lasts longer than 5 minutes, call an ambulance
   d. Once the seizure has stopped, roll the child onto their side

3. What are the indications for referral in general practice?

   Prolonged duration, focal seizure or other type of complex seizure, possible meningitis (meningism, petechial rash, altered consciousness, no obvious focus, under 18 months), abnormal neurology, cardiorespiratory compromise or parental anxiety, as will often be the case with the first febrile convulsion.

Case 2: epilepsy
Presentation
Adrian is a 3-year-old boy who has been brought in by his mum, having had a 5-minute 'fit'. He was sitting and watching television

at the time, then mum noticed he was lying down unconscious, with his arms and legs rhythmically jerking, and his eyes rolled back. She called an ambulance straight away and, after 5 minutes, the seizure stopped and he was noted to have passed urine and bitten his tongue. He was unconscious for a further 5 minutes, and both mum and the paramedics noted that he was very drowsy and confused for almost an hour and does not seem to remember the event. This is his first seizure; he is otherwise fit and well with no medical conditions and has had no recent infections. He was born at term by normal vaginal delivery after an uneventful pregnancy, weighing 3.8 kg, and was discharged home the same day. He had no issues in the neonatal period, is feeding well and has hit all of his developmental milestones. He is not on any medications and has no allergies, and immunizations are up to date. He lives at home with mum and dad, and there is no significant family history of epilepsy or seizure disorders or of any other illnesses. There are no smokers at home, no pets and no history of recent travel. Mum is worried about epilepsy or the possibility of a brain tumour.

In summary, this is a 3-year-old boy, normally fit and well, who presents with a history of a 5-minute tonic–clonic convulsion while watching television, associated with urinary incontinence, tongue biting, amnesia of the event and a post-ictal phase of an hour. These findings are consistent with a diagnosis of an epileptic generalized tonic–clonic seizure.

Other possible findings

1. Current episode: expiratory grunt at onset, observed tonic 'stiff' phase that normally lasts around 10 seconds, faecal incontinence.
2. Past medical history: complicated birth history, poor developmental milestone progression or learning disabilities, movement disorders.

Questions

(Answers based on current NICE guidelines)

1. What is epilepsy?

   Epilepsy is a neurological condition characterized by unprovoked recurrent epileptic seizures. An epileptic seizure is the clinical manifestation of abnormal and excessive discharge of a set of neurons in the brain. Epilepsy is not a single disease entity; rather, it is a symptom of a range of underlying neurological disorders.

2. How is epilepsy classified?

   The classification of epilepsy has undergone many changes over the last two decades. Earlier classifications used terms such as grand mal and petit mal seizures but these are no longer in use.

   More recently, epileptic seizures have been classified as 'generalized' and 'focal'.

   Generalized seizures arise within bilaterally distributed networks of the cerebral hemispheres, whereas focal seizures originate within networks limited to one cerebral hemisphere. Generalized seizures include tonic–clonic, absence (abrupt halt to current activity followed by a vacant stare and unresponsiveness), myoclonic (single brief jerks), clonic, tonic and atonic (abrupt loss of tone) seizures. Focal seizures are described according to the severity (with or without loss of consciousness) or according to their site of origin.

Infantile spasms (abrupt truncal flexion or extension with raised arms and legs in <1 year olds) are classified separately. It is important to recognize this entity as untreated it can lead to neuroregression and severe developmental delay.

The complete classification of epilepsy is undertaken and reviewed by the International League Against Epilepsy and fully incorporates the many different types of epilepsy.

3. What do you understand by the term 'epilepsy syndrome'?

Epilepsy syndromes are a combination of clinical and seizure characteristics, with a typical pattern, age of onset, electroencephalogram (EEG) and prognosis. An accurate diagnosis can ensure the correct treatment, monitoring and counselling for the parents. There are many epilepsy syndromes but two common syndromes are:
   a. Childhood absence epilepsy
      i. Age at onset: 4–10 years
      ii. Clinical: frequent absences (sudden onset and offset) lasting up to 20 seconds, normal development, family history
      iii. EEG: 3-Hz bilateral synchronous spike and wave discharges
      iv. Prognosis: tends to resolve in adolescence
   b. Benign rolandic epilepsy
      i. Age at onset: 4–10 years
      ii. Clinical: usually nocturnal seizures with unilateral numbness and twitching of the face lasting 1–2 minutes, may become generalized, normal development
      iii. EEG: centro-temporal spikes (relating to the rolandic area)
      iv. Prognosis: excellent prognosis with resolution in adolescence

4. How would you investigate this child and what is the role of EEG in the investigation of epilepsy?

A first fit in the absence of a fever should be investigated for an underlying cause, including blood glucose (hypoglycaemia), full blood count (infection), urea and electrolytes (electrolyte disturbance), calcium and magnesium. A 12-lead ECG must be done as cardiac syncopal episodes can be difficult to distinguish from epileptic fits, especially when a good history is difficult to obtain. No imaging, EEG or initiation of treatment would be indicated on first presentation with a generalized seizure in an otherwise well child with normal development, but the child would be referred to a paediatric neurologist/general paediatrician with a special interest in epilepsy for further assessment and monitoring. A MRI/CT head should be considered if the presenting complaint was a focal seizure as these could indicate an underlying structural lesion. However, focal seizures can be idiopathic.

The current NICE guidelines (2012) advise that an EEG should only be performed to support a clinical diagnosis of epilepsy and not used alone to make the diagnosis (note that approximately 5% of the normal population have abnormal EEG findings). If an EEG is considered necessary, it should be performed after the second epileptic seizure, though a specialist may choose to perform an EEG after the first seizure in certain circumstances. Importantly, a normal EEG does not rule out epilepsy.

An EEG can be helpful in determining the epilepsy syndrome, and this is useful for prognosis.

CLINICAL SCENARIO: BEDWETTING

Bedwetting, or enuresis, is a classic example of where a thorough history is the key to informing further management, whether that be simple measures for primary enuresis (e.g. enuresis alarms), psychosocial support (e.g. in bullying or sexual abuse), medications (e.g. laxatives in constipation) or specialized investigations (e.g. urodynamic studies). In England, it is estimated that 1 in 6 five-year-olds, 1 in 10 seven-year-olds and 1 in 14 ten-year-olds wet the bed at least twice a week; 1% of the population will have enuresis persisting into adulthood.

Typical findings in the history for common diagnoses include:

Diagnosis	Features on history
Physiological	
Primary enuresis (maturational)	Has never been dry
	Primarily nocturnal enuresis
	No pain or other symptoms
Inattention	Enuresis at any time of day
	Commoner in boys
	Common in children with ADHD
Constipation	Hard stools passed infrequently and with straining
	Poor fibre/fluid intake in diet
Pathological	
Urinary tract infection	Short history of dysuria, frequency, urgency and fever
	Unwell/off food
	May have suprapubic pain
Diabetes mellitus	Polyuria and polydipsia lead to increased need to void
	Thirst, weight loss, lethargy
Bladder dysfunction/overactive bladder	Persistent primary daytime enuresis
	Long history of urgency and frequency
	May be associated with pain

Continued

Diagnosis	Features on history
Congenital malformation, e.g. posterior urethral valves	Only in boys Problems with voiding from birth
Neurological disorder, e.g. spina bifida	History of neurological problems from birth May have cognitive impairment May also have incontinence of faeces
Psychosocial	Possible sources include the home (family relationships), school (bullying, performance) or sexual abuse

Case 1: primary enuresis

Presentation

Brian is an 8-year-old boy who has been brought in by mum with nocturnal enuresis that occurs about twice per week. He wakes up having wet the bed, has no pain or any other symptoms, has normal regular bowel movements and has never been dry. He is otherwise fit and well with no medical conditions, was born at term by normal vaginal delivery after an uneventful pregnancy, weighing 3.1 kg, and was discharged home the same day. He had no issues in the neonatal period. He has a good diet, and there are no developmental concerns. He enjoys school, plays on the football and cricket teams and is friends with most of his class. He is not on any medications, and immunizations are up to date. He lives at home with mum and dad and baby brother, who is 4 months old, and neither mum nor dad can remember bedwetting regularly at his age. There are no smokers at home, no pets and no history of recent travel. Mum and dad are supportive of Brian but are concerned for him as he is becoming more embarrassed and upset by these episodes and beginning to become withdrawn.

In summary, this is an 8-year-old boy with nocturnal enuresis in the absence of any other symptoms. These findings are consistent with a diagnosis of primary nocturnal enuresis.

Other possible findings

1. Current: daytime incontinence, diuretics/high fluid intake in the evenings.
2. Past medical history: family history, other elements of developmental delay.

Questions

(Answers based on current NICE guidelines)

1. How would you manage this child?

   Simple measures in primary nocturnal enuresis include:

   a. Ensure an adequate fluid intake and healthy diet but avoid excess fluid intake and caffeinated drinks in the evening
   b. Encourage the child to empty their bladder regularly during the day and before going to sleep and, if they wake, encourage them to use the toilet before going back to sleep

c. Ensuring easy access to a toilet, which in younger children might include a potty by the bedside

d. In the older child, it is also important to ask them if they can think of anything that might be contributing to the problem

e. A reward system, such as a 'star chart' can also be used for agreed behaviour rather than for dry nights, e.g. emptying the bladder before going to sleep

f. Not using penalty systems

   If these simple measures fail, further options include:

   i. First-line management is trial of an enuresis alarm for 4 weeks. If there is improvement, once a minimum of 14 consecutive dry nights have been achieved, the child can be trialled without the alarm.

   ii. If there is no improvement or if an alarm is inappropriate/ unacceptable to the child or family, in children over 7 years of age, desmopressin can be used. If there was some benefit with the alarm, the desmopressin can be trialled alongside the alarm. Fluids should be restricted from 1 hour before the dose to 8 hours after the dose.

   iii. If response remains unsatisfactory, refer to a specialist for consideration of anticholinergic or imipramine therapy.

2. What are the criteria for referral to secondary care with enuresis?

   NICE criteria for referral are:

   a. Severe daytime symptoms

   b. Symptoms and urinalysis suggestive of diabetes mellitus

   c. History of recurrent urinary tract infections (UTIs)

   d. Known or suspected physical or neurological problems

   e. Developmental, attention or learning difficulties

   f. Family problems or vulnerable child, young person or family

   g. Behavioural or emotional problems

   h. If no improvement with desmopressin, for consideration of anticholinergic/imipramine therapy

3. How might the history be different in a child with detrusor instability, and how might they be further investigated?

   The typical history in detrusor instability is long-standing diurnal enuresis with urinary frequency, urgency and staccato flow of urine. In some cases, there may additionally be perineal or suprapubic pain. A characteristic sign in young girls that might be noted by the parents is Vincent's curtsey sign, where the child crouches low down, pushing the heel into the perineum, in an attempt to augment the sphincter.

   Urge syndrome, which is also due to detrusor instability, typically presents with very small volumes of urine being lost, only enough to cause small damp patches.

These children should be referred to a specialist for further management. The gold standard of investigation for detrusor instability is urodynamic studies, which will show detrusor contractions during the filling phase while the patient is trying to inhibit voiding. However, urodynamic studies can be upsetting for the child and, in many cases, ultrasound of the renal tract with post-void residuals and simple urinary flow studies may be all that is required to make the diagnosis and inform management.

CLINICAL SCENARIO: HEADACHE

Headache is a common presenting complaint in school-age children, and most are benign in nature. However, there are a number of serious causes of headache in children, and it is important to take a thorough history to rule these out before you can safely discharge the child. It is useful to divide the causes between acute and chronic/recurrent, remembering that an acute headache may be the first presentation of a recurrent cause, e.g. first migraine, first tension headache etc.

Typical findings in the history for each diagnosis include:

Diagnosis	Features on history
Acute	
Meningitis	Fever and unwell Neck stiffness and photophobia May have purpuric rash if meningococcal
Blocked shunt	History of hydrocephalus with VP/VA shunt insertion Signs of raised intracranial pressure (ICP)
Intracranial bleed	May have precipitating trauma Signs of meningism and/or raised ICP Altered consciousness and/or neurological deficit
Referred pain	Sinusitis: facial pain and tenderness over maxillary sinuses Otitis media: ear pain and reduced hearing on that side Otitis externa: painful/itchy ears with discharge and reduced hearing Dental caries/abscess: poor dentition and nutrition, gum pain
Chronic/recurrent	
Tension headache	Generalized ache or band-like tightness over front of forehead Able to continue with daily activities No nausea or vomiting but may have mild photophobia
Migraine	Classically unilateral and pulsating, may be frontal Nausea, vomiting, photophobia and/or phonophobia Unable to continue with daily activities and aggravated by activity May be preceded by aura Family history
Raised intracranial pressure	Headache (±vomiting) typically worse in the morning Increasing frequency/severity from date of onset Seizures and/or weakness, diplopia, poor coordination Regression in developmental milestones/school performance

Case 1: migraine
Presentation

Nina is an 11-year-old girl who has been referred by her GP at mum's request, with a 4-month history of intermittent headaches, occurring between once and twice a month, with no symptoms between attacks. She describes them as a severe, throbbing pain on the left side of her head that make her feel sick, with vomiting on one occasion. The headaches can last up to 6 hours and settle with painkillers and lying down in a dark room, as light makes the headache worse. She is otherwise fit and well with no medical conditions. She was born at term by normal vaginal delivery after an uneventful pregnancy and was discharged home the same day. There were no developmental concerns growing up, and she has a healthy diet and is growing well and is doing well at school where she has several friends and is captain of the netball team. She is not on any medications, and immunizations are up to date. She lives at home with mum and dad and her 15-year-old brother, all of whom are well, though mum remembers having similar terrible headaches as a teenager, which eventually disappeared. There are no smokers at home, no pets and no history of recent travel. Her parents are concerned because she has been sent home from school on three occasions as the pain has been so severe; they are worried that there might be a serious underlying cause.

In summary, this is an 11-year-old girl, normally fit and well, presenting with recurrent headaches that are severe, unilateral and throbbing in nature, associated with nausea, vomiting, photophobia, inability to continue with daily activities and a maternal history of similar headaches. These findings are consistent with a diagnosis of migraine (without aura).

Other possible findings

Current: bilateral or frontal headache, or starts unilateral and spreads to other side, phonophobia, lightheadedness, abdominal cramps, premonitory phase preceding headache (e.g. changes in mood, appetite, thirst), aura (most commonly visual aura, e.g. blurring or fortification spectra), postdromal fatigue, trigger factors (see below).

Questions

1. What are common triggers for migraines?

   Trigger factors are only found in a minority of migraine sufferers, and a migraine diary can help to identify them. In these individuals, avoidance of these triggers can prevent the onset of migraines and improve quality of life, though good quality evidence on this is lacking. Common triggers identified by patients include:

   a. Physiological: stress, hunger, dehydration, fatigue, lack of sleep and hormonal triggers, including menstruation.

   b. Dietary: cheese, chocolate, alcohol, citrus fruits and products containing tyramine and MSG.

2. What are the criteria for diagnosing migraine without aura and how do they differ from the criteria for a tension-type headache?

The International Headache Society (IHS) criteria for the diagnosis of migraine without aura (formerly common migraine) are:

a. At least FIVE headache attacks lasting 1–72 hours (4–72 hours in adults), with at least TWO of:
   i. Unilateral or bilateral
   ii. Throbbing/pulsating quality
   iii. Moderate or severe intensity (inhibits or prohibits daily activities)
   iv. Aggravated by routine physical activity
b. During the headache at least ONE of:
   i. Phonophobia and/or photophobia
   ii. Nausea and/or vomiting

The IHS criteria for diagnosing tension-type headache are:

a. Headache lasting from 30 minutes to 7 days
b. At least TWO of:
   i. Pressing/tightening (non-pulsatile) quality
   ii. Mild or moderate intensity (may inhibit, but does not prohibit activity)
   iii. Bilateral location
   iv. No aggravation by walking up stairs or similar routine physical activity
c. BOTH of:
   i. No nausea or vomiting (anorexia may occur)
   ii. Photophobia and phonophobia are absent, or one but not both are present

3. How would you manage this patient?

The management of migraine should take a four-step approach:

a. Explain and reassure
   i. Migraine is the most common cause of recurrent headache in children
   ii. It does not reflect any underlying serious pathology, e.g. brain tumour
   iii. Attacks can be managed, and severity and frequency can be reduced
   iv. Generally, migraine improves with age
b. Identify and avoid possible trigger factors
   i. A headache diary can be used to identify possible trigger factors, while making clear that trigger factors are only found in a minority of patients
   ii. General advice regarding sleep hygiene, reducing stress, good diet and regular fluids may all help to reduce severity
c. Relieve symptoms during an acute attack
   i. Non-pharmacological advice for dealing with an attack includes lying in a cool, dark room and encouraging sleep

ii. First-line treatment includes simple analgesics such as paracetamol or ibuprofen early in the attack, with advice about medication over-use headache (MOH)

iii. If simple analgesics fail to control the pain, in children over 12, sumatriptan nasal spray can be used

iv. If nausea and vomiting are troubling symptoms, domperidone can be used in all ages and prochlorperazine can be used in children over 12

d. Prophylaxis

i. Prophylactic therapy should be considered in cases such as this, where migraine attacks are interfering with school attendance or other important aspects of the child's life

ii. First-line options include beta-blockers or pizotifen, though there is little evidence for efficacy in children

iii. Second-line options that can be prescribed by a specialist include topiramate, sodium valproate or amitryptyline

Case 2: raised intracranial pressure
Presentation

Becky is an 8-year-old girl who has been referred by her GP at mum's request, with a 1-month history of worsening headaches. She describes them as worst first thing in the morning, and last week she has also vomited in the morning on two occasions. The headaches ease by lunchtime, she has no neck stiffness or photophobia and her vision is normal. She is otherwise fit and well with no medical conditions. She was born at term by normal vaginal delivery after an uneventful pregnancy and was discharged home the same day. There were no developmental concerns growing up, she has a healthy diet and is growing well and is popular at school and doing well academically. She is not on any medications and immunizations are up to date. She lives at home with mum and dad, both of whom are well, and there is no family history of headaches. There are no smokers at home, no pets and no history of recent travel. Her parents are concerned because the headaches are not getting better, the vomiting is getting worse and they are worried about a serious underlying cause.

In summary, this is an 8-year-old girl, normally fit and well, presenting with a 1-month history of worsening headaches that are most severe in the morning, now associated with vomiting. These findings are consistent with a diagnosis of a raised intracranial pressure headache.

Other possible findings

Current: headache worse on coughing, straining or moving head, neck stiffness, new onset seizures, abnormalities of gait or coordination, changes in mental state including lethargy, irritability, change in personality or deteriorating school performance and double vision. Late symptoms include motor weakness and decreased conscious level.

Questions

1. What are the possible causes for raised ICP in this child?

    The differential diagnosis for raised ICP in children includes cerebral tumour, hydrocephalus, benign intracranial hypertension and cerebral abscess (though the absence of fever or predisposing illness such as congenital heart disease, meningitis or septicaemia in this case makes an abscess unlikely). The most common cause overall is traumatic brain injury, though the history here is inconsistent with that diagnosis and there are also rarer causes such as cerebral venous sinus thrombosis.

    The time course and presentation in this child are highly suspicious for a cerebral tumour.

2. What features would you look for on examination of this child and how would you further investigate the cause of the headache?

    Classically, the triad of raised ICP is headache, vomiting and papilloedema, so fundoscopy should be performed looking for blurring of the disc margin, loss of venous pulsation and flame-shaped haemorrhages. A full neurological examination should also be performed, looking for visual field defects, weakness, abnormal gait and coordination, irregular pupil size, diplopia and cranial nerve III and VI nerve palsies.

    This child would need to be urgently imaged with contrast CT/MRI head (the preferred imaging is MRI).

3. What are the common types of brain tumour in children?

    The common types of brain tumour are: astrocytoma (~45%), embryonal tumours including primitive neuroectodermal tumour and medulloblastoma (~20%) and ependymoma (~10%).

COMMUNICATION SKILLS IN PAEDIATRICS

Explanation of why immunization is important to a mother

'You are a FY1 doctor in paediatrics. James is a 6-month-old boy who was admitted with viral gastroenteritis and has now recovered and is ready to be discharged home. During the initial clerking, it was noted that James is not immunized. You have been asked to discuss immunizations with the mother prior to discharge.'

Score Sheet

Scores: 1 = Not attempted; 2 = Attempted, unsatisfactory; 3 = Attempted, satisfactory

Action	1	2	3
1. Introduces self, checks the patient's details and develops rapport			
2. Clarifies history regarding immunization			
3. Elicits mother's ideas and concerns regarding immunizations			

Continued

Action	1	2	3
4. Explains role and importance of immunizations			
5. Answers common questions regarding immunizations			
6. Checks understanding and provides written information			
7. Summarizes and closes appropriately			
Overall score	/21		

1. Begin every communication skills station by introducing yourself and confirming that you are speaking to the right person by checking the patient's name and date of birth and the relationship of the carer to the patient. In this scenario, it would also be important to establish whether there are any other siblings to check if there are other unimmunized children at home; this will also help to build rapport.

2. Regardless of the details in the vignette, remember to clarify the history of the presenting complaint yourself. This will both provide a context for the discussion and help to build rapport:

   I understand that James was admitted for a tummy bug and he's now better. We routinely ask all parents about the immunizations that their children might have had; may I ask whether James has had any immunizations?

3. In order to pitch the explanation appropriately, you should always elicit the carer's understanding and concerns regarding immunizations before explaining their role and importance:

   May I ask you what you understand by the term immunizations? ... What are your main worries or concerns that have led you to not get James immunized?

   Common reasons for not getting children vaccinated include:
   a. My child is healthy so why should he have an injection?
   b. The diseases are so rare that he'll probably never get them anyway.
   c. I'm worried about the risk of autism and other diseases.
   d. His sister had a reaction to one of her jabs, so I didn't give him any.
   e. I'm worried that he will get the infection after the jab.

4. Remember when explaining medical scenarios, always use simple, clear, jargon-free language. An example of how to explain the role and importance of immunizations would be:

   The diseases that we immunize against can be very serious for both children and adults, in some cases leading to long-term disability or death.

   An immunization jab contains a vaccine, which is an inactive form of the bacteria or virus that causes the infection. Because it is inactive, your child cannot get the infection from the jab. However, it still stimulates the body's immune system to develop immunity from that infection. In this way, if your child is ever exposed to the infection, their body can fight it off before it develops, so they won't become unwell or develop any long-term complications.

Although these diseases have become rare since the advent of immunizations, more recently the immunization rates have fallen and some of these diseases are beginning to reappear, in particular measles and whooping cough. This has made it even more important to be up to date with immunizations.

5. Common follow-up questions and sample answers include:

Q: What about the risk of autism?

A: There has been a lot in the media about the MMR vaccine and autism following a study published in 1998 by Dr Andrew Wakefield. He claimed that his initial findings suggested a link between the MMR vaccine and autism and bowel disease. However, his work, which was based on 12 patients, has been completely discredited and retracted from the journals, and he has been struck off the medical register for it. Further studies performed since then, including a study on more than half a million Danish children, have shown no link between MMR and autism.

Q: What if his sister had a reaction to her first injection?

A: In that case, there is no reason why the child cannot have the immunization. The only two reasons why a child would not be able to have an immunization are if the child himself has had a severe reaction to an immunization, e.g. difficulty breathing, or if the child's immune system is weakened, e.g. if they are on treatment for cancer. You can always speak to your GP or practice nurse if you are concerned that either of these may be the case.

Q: Are these illnesses really that serious?

A: Yes; some of these diseases can cause a very serious illness and others, which may be milder, can have very serious complications and may be fatal. Some serious complications of diseases that we vaccinate against include:

Disease	Complications
Measles	Pneumonia, meningitis, encephalitis, hepatitis
Mumps	Orchitis, pancreatitis, meningitis, encephalitis, deafness
Rubella	Congenital rubella syndrome leads to multiple defects in fetuses exposed in the first trimester
Pertussis	Pneumonia, seizures, brain damage
Diphtheria	Respiratory failure, myocarditis, diaphragmatic paralysis
Haemophilus B	Pneumonia, meningitis, epiglottitis
Tetanus	Tetanus itself causes muscle spasms and stiffness, complications include sudden cardiac death, PE, aspiration pneumonia and rhabdomyolysis

Continued

Disease	Complications
Polio	Polio itself causes a meningitis-like illness and can lead to wasting of the muscles, flaccid paralysis of the limbs and difficulty breathing
Meningitis C	Meningitis and septicaemia
Pneumococcal disease	Pneumonia, meningitis, septicaemia
Human papillomavirus (HPV)	Cervical cancer, head and neck cancer

Q: They haven't caught any of these infections in their first 6 months, so maybe they just have a strong immunity and can fight off the infections anyway?

A: Newborn babies have immunity to several diseases that the mother is immune to because antibodies pass from the mother to the baby via the placenta. This immunity is called passive immunity, and it wanes over the first few months to the first year, leaving the baby susceptible to the diseases. Immunization provides what we call active immunity and provides long-term immunity.

Q: How many injections do they have to have?

A: The UK routine immunization schedule (as of November 2014) is as follows:

Timing	Immunization (each injection on a separate line)
2 months old	DTaP/IPV/Hib PCV Rotavirus
3 months old	DTaP/IPV/Hib MenC Rotavirus
4 months old	DTaP/IPV/Hib PCV
12–13 months old	Hib/MenC MMR PCV
2, 3 and 4 years old	Children's flu vaccine
3 years, and 4 months–5 years old	DTaP/IPV booster MMR
Girls 12–13 years old	HPV (two injections between 6 months to 2 years apart)
13–15 years old	MenC booster
13–18 years old	Td/IPV booster

DTaP = diphtheria, tetanus and acellular pertussis; Td = tetanus and diphtheria; IPV = inactivated poliovirus vaccine; Hib = haemophilus influenza type B; PCV = pneuomococcal vaccine; MenC = meningitis C; MMR = measles, mumps and rubella; HPV = human papillomavirus vaccine.

Your GP or midwife will advise you if further immunizations are recommended, e.g. hepatitis B or the BCG vaccine for tuberculosis. These will be recommended if you come from or live in a high-risk area for these diseases.

6. Having answered the mother's questions, it is important that you check that she has understood your explanation and answers and that you clarify any details on which she is not clear.

All the information provided during a consultation can be a lot to take in; therefore, it is important to provide that information in a written leaflet. Explain to the mother that it contains the information that you have discussed today and that it lists a Web site and phone number that she can call for further advice on the matter.

7. Summarize the discussion that you have had, including:
   a. The mother's concerns
   b. Your explanation of the importance of immunizations
   c. The questions that you have answered

Close the consultation by once again checking whether the mother has any further questions, advising that the parents can arrange for their GP to complete the course of immunizations if they decide that they would like to proceed with this, thanking her and then saying goodbye.

Explain to a mother/child how to use an inhaler and peak flow meter

'You are a FY1 doctor in paediatrics. Tom is a 7-year-old boy who presented with bilateral wheeze and difficulty breathing for the first time this winter and is now ready to be discharged home. Before he goes, he and his mum need to be shown how to use the salbutamol inhaler and spacer that he has just been prescribed and how to use the peak flow meter to keep a peak flow diary to take to his GP in 2 weeks' time. The mother has been given an inhaler plan for the number of puffs and timing of the inhaler.'

Score Sheet

Scores: 1 = Not attempted; 2 = Attempted, unsatisfactory; 3 = Attempted, satisfactory

Action	1	2	3
1. Introduces self, checks the patient's details and develops rapport			
2. Clarifies history of presenting complaint			
3. Establishes mother's/child's ideas and concerns regarding how to use an inhaler/spacer			
4. Explains how to use inhaler/spacer to mother and child			
5. Explains how to use peak flow meter and peak flow diary			
6. Answers common follow-up questions appropriately			
7. Checks understanding and provides written information			
8. Summarizes and closes appropriately			
Overall score		/24	

1. Begin every communication skills station by introducing yourself and confirming that you are speaking to the right person by checking the

patient's name and date of birth and the relationship of the carer to the patient.

2. Regardless of the details in the vignette, remember to clarify the history of the presenting complaint yourself. This will provide a context for the discussion and help to build rapport:

> *Can you tell me a little bit about what brought Tom into hospital today? ... Has he ever had anything like this before?*

3. In order to pitch the explanation of how to use the inhaler and spacer device appropriately, it is important to first elicit the child and mother's existing understanding and any specific concerns they may have. The child may have used inhalers in the past with poor technique, or the mother may have experience from another child at home with asthma:

> *Has Tom ever used an inhaler before or have you ever been shown how to use one in the past? ... Is there any aspect that you're particularly concerned about?*

4. The most commonly used inhalers are pressurized metered dose inhalers (MDIs), where each dose is released as a 'puff' by pressing on top of the inhaler. The other main group of inhalers are breath-activated inhalers, which do not require you to push down on a canister, instead releasing the dose when you breathe in sharply. There are several types of breath-activated inhalers, e.g. breath-activated MDIs and dry powder inhalers, but they tend not to be suitable for young children as a strong breath is required to trigger the dose.

    Therefore, the most common type of inhaler you will need to explain in an OSCE is the pressurized MDI. Because children under the age of 12 tend not to be able to coordinate pushing down the canister and breathing in, they are always prescribed with a spacer.

    There are several different spacers available, the most common being the Aerochamber Plus® system; they are available in different sizes with masks for younger children and mouthpieces for older children. Accordingly, you may need to adapt the dialogue to suit the age of the child; remember to address both mother and child using appropriate language.

> *Tom's symptoms indicate that he may have asthma and that is why he has been prescribed the inhaler. The inhaler releases a medication called salbutamol into his lungs, which opens up his airways and makes it easier for him to breathe.*
>
> *The inhaler is just a plastic casing with a canister inside, and when you push down on the canister, it releases the medication with a 'puff'. Because it's difficult for children to push down on the canister and breathe in at exactly the right time, the inhaler has to be attached to this spacer in order for the medication to get to the lungs to work properly.*

The correct way to use the inhaler and spacer is as follows:
(Demonstrate to the child/mum as appropriate in tandem with the description.)

1. *Look at the spacer to make sure that there are no loose parts or small objects inside*
2. *Remove the cap from the inhaler and the spacer*
3. *Shake the inhaler before each use*
4. *Insert the inhaler into the backpiece of the spacer*
5. *Put the mouthpiece of the inhaler in your mouth to ensure an effective seal*
6. *Push down the canister once*
7. *Breathe in and out through the mouthpiece five times*
8. *While you are breathing, if you hear a whistle, then you are breathing too hard*
9. *Remove the mouthpiece from your mouth*
10. *Wait 30 seconds, shake the inhaler again and then repeat according to the asthma plan that you have*

Once you have explained and demonstrated how to use the inhaler/spacer, check that the parent and child have understood by asking them to show you what you have just demonstrated. This is good practice generally and part of the BTS/SIGN guidelines.

5. Although trial of treatment is the preferred 'investigation' of children with likely or suspected asthma, serial peak expiratory flow readings can also support the diagnosis and may be used in older children alongside the trial of treatment. In these cases, the child and carer have to be shown how to use the peak flow meter and how to record the results in a peak flow diary. Remember to demonstrate appropriately throughout:

This is called a peak flow meter, and when you blow into it, it measures the fastest speed that you can blow air out of your lungs. It is important that you use it properly so that you can compare the results at different times. The proper way to use it is as follows:

1. *Put the marker on the peak flow meter to '0'*
2. *Hold the peak flow meter horizontally*
3. *Take a deep breath in*
4. *Seal your lips around the mouthpiece*
5. *Blow out as hard and as fast as you can into the device*
6. *Take a few normal breaths, and then take two further readings*
7. *Record the best reading*

If the three readings are not similar, your technique may not be quite right. The most common errors are not sealing your lips around the mouthpiece properly and not blowing as hard as you can. It often helps to try to think about it as trying to get all of the air out of your lungs in the shortest possible time.

(Demonstrate how to use the peak flow meter once you have explained it, then check that the parent and child have understood by asking the child to use it and giving supportive advice as appropriate.)

The results should be recorded in the peak flow diary like this: by drawing dots or crosses next to the best reading, morning and evening, over a 2-week period. In asthma, we often see that the reading is higher in the evening than in the morning, so you might get a sawtooth pattern. You should then take this diary to your GP, who will be able to advise you as to whether further treatment or monitoring would be appropriate.

(Demonstrate how to plot one or two readings, and then check that the parent and child have understood by asking the child to plot another one or two readings, again offering supportive advice as appropriate.)

6. Common follow-up questions and sample answers include:

Q: What is asthma and how has he got it?

A: (You may wish to offer to draw a picture to assist with this explanation.) When we breathe in, the air enters our nose and mouth, travels down our windpipe and then enters the lungs via smaller and smaller branching airways. People with asthma are susceptible to inflammation of these small airways in the lungs. When this happens, the airways become much narrower because the muscles tighten and phlegm can be produced, which can block some of the airways. This makes it difficult to breathe, leading to shortness of breath, 'wheezy' breathing and coughing.

We don't know for sure what causes asthma. We do know that it is more common in children with a family history of asthma, eczema, hay fever or allergies or if the child themselves suffers from these. We also know that smoking during pregnancy increases the risk of the child suffering from asthma.

Q: Is there anything to watch out for that could make it worse?

A: Asthma affects different people in different ways. In some people, it may flare up for no apparent reason. In others, there may be certain 'triggers' that make it worse. Common triggers include: pollen, colds and chest infections, cigarette smoke, cold, animals and exercise. Importantly, exercise is good for you if you have asthma; it may just be that you need to take an inhaler before you start exercising.

Q: I had it when I was younger and grew out of it, so does that mean that he will grow out of it too?'

A: Some children with asthma do 'grow out of it' as they become adults, and some find that their symptoms become much milder, for example, only occurring when they pick up an infection. However, some children will continue to have asthma into adulthood, and it is impossible to predict which of these groups your child will fall into.

7. Having answered the mother's questions, it is important that you check that she has understood your explanation and answers and to clarify any details on which she is not clear.

All the information provided during a consultation can be a lot to take in; therefore, it is important to provide that information in a written leaflet. Explain to the mother that it contains the information that you have discussed today and that it has a Web site and phone number that she can call for further advice on the matter.

8. Summarize the discussion that you have had, including:
   a. The mother's concerns
   b. Your explanation of how to use the inhaler/spacer
   c. The questions that you have answered

Close the consultation by once again checking whether the mother has any further questions, thanking them both and then saying goodbye.

Explain to a mother why a child who has accidentally ingested paracetamol suspension has to be kept in for at least 4 hours

'You are a FY1 doctor in paediatrics. Jane, a 4-year-old girl, has presented having drunk some Calpol that was left unattended on the kitchen counter. She swallowed the Calpol 3 hours ago, has been reviewed by one of the paediatric registrars and has been well and running around since. Mum would like to take her home now. Explain why she cannot leave until the child has had a blood paracetamol level taken and advise her that a health visitor will be visiting tomorrow to talk to the family as a routine follow-up.'

Score Sheet

Scores: 1 = Not attempted; 2 = Attempted, unsatisfactory; 3 = Attempted, satisfactory

Action	1	2	3
1. Introduces self, checks the patient's details and develops rapport			
2. Clarifies history of presenting complaint			
3. Establishes mother's ideas and concerns about paracetamol ingestion			
4. Explains the reason why the child cannot leave hospital			
5. Answers common questions about paracetamol ingestion appropriately			
6. Advises mother that a health visitor will be visiting			
7. Checks mother's understanding and provides written information			
8. Summarizes and closes appropriately			
Overall score		/24	

1. Begin every communication skills station by introducing yourself and confirming that you are speaking to the right person by checking the patient's name and date of birth and the relationship of the carer to the patient.

2. Regardless of the details in the vignette, remember to clarify the history of presenting complaint yourself. This will provide a context for the discussion and help to build rapport, e.g.:

Can you tell me a little bit about why you've brought Jane in to see us today? ... Do you know how much Calpol she might have drunk?

3. In order to pitch the explanation of paracetamol ingestion appropriately, it is important to first elicit the mother's understanding and her specific concerns, which will be informed by her initial discussion with the registrar who first saw the child, e.g.:

Can I ask what you've already been told about the risks associated with swallowing Calpol and what we need to do next? ... Is there anything specifically that you're worried about?

The mother may have been told about the need to have a blood test at 4 hours but not fully understand the reason why. Commonly in these scenarios, the mother will have some reason why she has to leave, such as picking up another child from school. In this situation, it is important that you help her to problem-solve, e.g. by asking her if a partner or friend can see to the other child, or if a teacher at school can keep an eye on the child in an after-school club. As a last resort, the mother can sometimes leave the patient at hospital to go and pick up another child and bring him or her there, but it is preferable for mothers to remain with young children.

4. Based upon the mother's prior understanding, explain the risks of paracetamol poisoning and the reason why the child has to stay in for the blood test. Remember, as with all explanation stations, use simple, jargon-free language and maintain eye contact to assess whether she understands what you are saying. In this case, because you are explaining that the consequences of paracetamol overdose are potentially very serious, you should take particular care with your tone of voice and body language to reassure her, and use appropriate pauses to allow her to ask questions as needed, e.g.:

Calpol contains the painkiller paracetamol. As with all medications, at the recommended dose it is safe and the risk of side effects is low. However, exceeding the recommended dose can in some cases lead to serious complications, including damage to the liver and kidneys.

In order to assess how much paracetamol Jane has ingested, we have to take a blood test 4 hours after she drank from the bottle. The reason that we have to wait 4 hours is because during this time the paracetamol is being absorbed into her system and, if we do the test too soon, we will underestimate the amount.

When we do this blood test, we will also send off her blood to check her liver and kidneys. When the results come back, if the levels are low, you can go home straight away. However, if the level is high, we will have to give her some medication through a drip to protect her system from the effects of the paracetamol. This treatment will last for 24 hours, so she would have to stay in overnight.

5. Common follow-up questions and answers include:

Q: But if she's so well now, doesn't that mean that she hasn't swallowed too much?

A: Children and adults who have had a paracetamol overdose can have no symptoms at all in the first 24 hours, though some may have some nausea and vomiting. The excess paracetamol starts to affect the liver after the first 24 hours and affects the kidneys later than this. Therefore, the only way to know how much paracetamol has been swallowed is to do the blood test after 4 hours.

Q: If it's so serious, shouldn't you do something now to get it out?

A: In adults and older children, when the paracetamol has been taken less than 1 hour before coming to hospital, it is possible to give something called 'activated charcoal'. This binds the paracetamol in the stomach and prevents it being absorbed by the body. However, when more than 1 hour has passed, the charcoal will not have enough of a chance to bind the paracetamol and so will be ineffective. Additionally, young children do not tolerate drinking the charcoal, which is quite unpleasant, and tend to vomit, so it is rarely used in this age group.

Q: How do you know if the level that comes back is too high?

A: We have a standardized graph called a 'nomogram' on which we plot the drug level. If the level is below the treatment line, we don't need to treat and, if it is above, we do need to treat.

6. Most units will arrange to have a health visitor visit the family after an accidental overdose in a child, simply to check that the child is well and to answer any follow-up questions and to check that the medicine cabinet is out of reach of the children. When explaining this to the mother, it is important to stress that this is routine and nobody is suggesting that there is any fault, e.g.:

Once we have discharged children who have come in with accidental poisoning, we always arrange for the health visitor to visit them at home. This is done mainly so that we can check that they are well from the incident and so that parents have a chance to ask any follow-up questions. The health visitor will also just check that the medicine cabinet is out of reach of the children and offer any appropriate advice. Over half of all poisonings occur in children under the age of 5, almost all of which are accidental; so this is just a routine action that we take to reduce the risk of future accidental poisoning.

7. Having answered the mother's questions, it is important that you check that she has understood your explanation and answers and clarify any details on which she is not clear.

All the information provided during a consultation can be a lot to take in; therefore, it is important to provide that information in a written leaflet. Explain to the mother that it contains the information that you have discussed today and that it has a Web site and phone number that she can call for further advice on the matter.

8. Summarize the discussion that you have had, including:
   a. The mother's concerns
   b. Your explanation of the importance of staying in for the blood test
   c. The questions that you have answered
   Close the consultation by once again checking whether the mother has any further questions, advising her that somebody will come to take the blood test at the appropriate time and that you will inform her of the result as soon as it is back. Remember to thank her before saying goodbye.

Advise a mother with regard to her questions about her 15-year-old son's treatment

'You are a FY1 doctor in paediatrics. James, a 15-year-old boy, presented last week with a sexually transmitted infection and was discharged with a course of antibiotics and appropriate follow-up. There was no suspicion of abuse, and his 15-year-old girlfriend was also treated. His mother has found the antibiotic tablets with the name of hospital on it and has come in to ask why they were prescribed. Advise her appropriately.'

Score Sheet

Scores: 1 = Not attempted; 2 = Attempted, unsatisfactory; 3 = Attempted, satisfactory

Action	1	2	3
1. Introduces self, checks personal details and develops rapport			
2. Establishes what parent already knows			
3. Explains the law on confidentiality using appropriate language			
4. Answers common follow-up questions appropriately			
5. Provides leaflet and checks understanding			
6. Summarizes and closes			
Overall score	/18		

1. Begin every communication skills station by introducing yourself and confirming that you are speaking to the right person by checking the patient's name and date of birth and the relationship of the carer to the patient.

2. Regardless of the details in the vignette, remember to elicit what the mother already knows yourself. This will both provide a context for the discussion and help to build rapport. It is particularly important to check whether the mother has spoken to her son about the antibiotics already and, if so, what he has told her and, if not, why not:

   Can I ask what you've already been told, either by James or by anybody else? … Have you spoken to James about this at all?

3. Regardless of whether the patient has spoken to his mother or not, you have a duty of confidentiality towards him. This means that he has the right to expect that no information about him will be disclosed to anybody, including his parents, without his consent. Note that this duty of confidentiality is both part of the GMC professional code of conduct and a legal obligation enshrined in case law. Consent is implied for discussions between health professionals as part of the patient's care.

   If the mother has not already spoken to her son, the first piece of advice would be for her to do so.

   If she has already spoken to her son and wants further information, or her son has refused to speak to her, then apologize for the fact that you cannot give her any information and explain why this is the case. Remember to use simple, jargon-free language and to maintain good eye contact and body language. It is particularly important in this scenario to keep the mother calm and explain that it is in her son's best interests to keep your duty of confidentiality towards him:

   I'm sorry, but by law I'm not actually able to discuss any details of James' care with anybody without his consent and that extends to you as a parent. He is 15 years old and competent to make his own decisions about his care. The law on confidentiality exists to maintain trust between doctors and patients – if teenagers felt that they could not trust doctors, then they would not come to see us with medical problems that could potentially be serious. My suggestion would therefore be for you to discuss this further directly with him.

4. You can be sure that the mother will have a few follow-up questions! Some common questions and answers include:

   Q: But he's only 15 years old and I'm his mother – you have to tell me what these antibiotics are for.

   A: While children are deemed legally able to make decisions about their treatment at the age of 16, they can do this at a younger age if they are competent to do so. This means that if they are able to understand and retain information, weigh up the risks and benefits, understand the consequences and arrive at a choice, then they are competent to make their own decisions. We always advise children to involve their parents, but we cannot force them to do so, and we cannot break their confidence without their consent.

   Q: Are you saying that there are no circumstances under which you can break the confidentiality of a 15-year-old boy?

   A: Under certain circumstances we can break confidentiality, but it is a difficult balance. First, if there is an overriding public interest; for example, if there is any risk of physical or sexual abuse, any risk of serious harm to themselves or others. Second, if the child does not have capacity to consent and third, under specific circumstances that are required by law, such as if they are involved in a road traffic collision. None of these circumstances apply here.

Q: Can I speak to your senior about this?

A: You can absolutely speak to one of my seniors when they are available. However, they will tell you the same thing because the duty of confidentiality is both part of the doctors' code of practice and part of English law. The best thing to do would be to speak to your son further about this.

5. Having answered the mother's questions, it is important that you check that she has understood your explanation and answers and clarify any details on which she is not clear.

It is important to provide the information on the law on confidentiality and children in a written leaflet. Explain to the mother that it contains the information that you have discussed today and that it has a Web site and phone number that she can call for further advice on the matter.

6. Summarize the discussion that you have had, including:
   a. The mother's concerns
   b. Your explanation of confidentiality
   c. The questions that you have answered

Close the consultation by once again checking whether the mother has any further questions and either advising her that you will go and ask your senior to come and see her, or thanking her and saying goodbye.

PAEDIATRIC EXAMINATION

General tips
Communicating with children

It is important to consider how to communicate with a child as thought processes vary with age. A child's development can be divided into three stages of life: preschool (2–5 years), school age (6–11 years) and adolescent (12–18 years), as illustrated in the table below.

Preschool	School age	Adolescent
Objects are alive, e.g. when a child bangs into a door they may remark that 'the door hurt me'	Beginning to solve problems	Developing wider social concerns, e.g. 'Should we be doing more to help third-world countries?'
Pretend play, e.g. 'my toys are leaving teddy out and he is sad'	Able to empathize with other peoples' views	Seeks independence from parents
Centre of their world, e.g. 'when I am asleep everyone else is asleep'	Becomes concerned about the future, e.g. 'Will I be picked for the netball team?'	
World is viewed from the child's perspective, e.g. 'when I close my eyes, Dad goes away'		

Therefore, a preschool child is more likely to respond to open rather than closed questions, to toys and puppets and the use of questions within their experience. A school-age child will respond to experiences they may have had, for example at school. An adolescent may wish the history and examination to be conducted without the parents present.

Introductions

Introduce yourself to the parents and child and explain the purpose of the examination. It is important to take the age of the child into account and the positioning of the child should be adapted accordingly. Babies may be examined on a bed with the parents nearby, and toddlers may be more cooperative while playing or sitting on their parent's lap. School-age children are more cooperative but may be concerned about privacy. Therefore younger children should be undressed to their underwear, and one should be more sensitive to exposure in older children.

Paediatric life support

'You see a collapsed child at an outdoor fete. Assuming the child is not responsive, please undertake basic paediatric life support on the mannequin provided. Finally, demonstrate the recovery position on the actor.'

Score Sheet

Scores: 1 = Not attempted; 2 = Attempted, unsatisfactory; 3 = Attempted, satisfactory

Action	1	2	3
1. Assesses for danger			
2. Aims to elicit a response			
3. Requests help			
4. Assesses and manages airway			
5. Assesses and manages breathing (rescue breaths)			
6. Assesses and manages circulation (chest compressions)			
7. States when cardiopulmonary resuscitation should stop			
8. Demonstrates the recovery position			
Overall score		/24	

For this station, you can use the DRS ABC approach (Danger, Response, Shout for help, Airway, Breathing, Circulation) as follows:

1. **Danger.** Assess the surrounding area for danger before approaching the child.
2. **Response.** Ask the child 'Are you alright?' DO NOT shake a child if you suspect that they may have a cervical injury. If the child responds, leave the child in the position that you found them if possible and get help if needed. Ensure that you reassess the child regularly.

3. **Shout for help** if the child is unresponsive.
4. **Airway.** If the child is unresponsive, turn the child onto their back (again, assuming there is no risk of spinal fracture). Open the airway using the head-tilt chin-lift manoeuvre. Place one hand on the child's forehead and, while placing the fingertips of the other under the chin, gently tilt the head back. Take care not to push too hard on the soft tissues from underneath as this pressure may block the airway. In infants (up to 1 year), the head should be in a neutral (flat) position. In older children, the head should be in the 'sniffing the morning air' position, similar to adults. Try a jaw thrust if this is not successful. A jaw thrust is achieved by placing two fingers of each hand behind the mandible and pushing the jaw anteriorly.
5. **Breathing.** Look for chest movements, listen for breath sounds and feel for breaths on your cheek for NO MORE THAN 10 SECONDS. If the child is breathing normally, but they are unconscious, then put them in the recovery position (see below) and get help if it has not already arrived. If the child is not breathing, five rescue breaths should be given. In infants, this is performed by placing your mouth over the nose and mouth. In older children, pinch the nose and give mouth-to-mouth resuscitation. The chest should rise with each breath if the rescue breaths are effective. If there is difficulty giving a good breath, open the mouth and attempt to remove any obvious obstruction. A blind finger sweep should never be performed.
6. **Circulation.** Check for a carotid pulse (if <1 year old, feel for a brachial pulse), for NO MORE THAN 10 SECONDS. The femoral pulse is an alternative location for palpation in all age groups. If there is a pulse, continue rescue breaths until the child is breathing on their own and then place the child in the recovery position if they are still unconscious. If there is no pulse after this time or the heart rate is <60 beats per minute, give chest compressions. In infants encircle the thorax with your hands, with your thumbs at the base of the sternum. In a small child, use the heel of the hand over the lower third of the sternum, keep your arm straight and apply pressure from vertically above the child. In older children, use both hands, with fingers interlocked over the lower third of the sternum. Again, keep your arms straight and apply pressure from vertically above the child. The compressions should be given at a rate of 100 beats per minute, aiming to depress the sternum by one-third the depth of the chest, at a ratio of 15 compressions to two breaths.
7. **Continue resuscitation until** there is spontaneous return of circulation, further help arrives or you become exhausted.
8. **Recovery position.** The following principles should be followed. The child should be placed in a lateral position to allow fluid to drain from the mouth and to prevent the tongue from falling backwards and causing airway obstruction. In infants, this may necessitate the use of pillows or blankets to maintain this position. The airway should be accessible and visible at all times. In older children, the adult recovery position can be used. Straighten both of the child's legs. Place the arm nearest

to you at right angles to the body. Bend the elbow with the palm facing upwards. Bring the other arm across the chest and place the back of the hand against the cheek nearest to you. Grasp the leg farthest from you above the knee and pull it upwards. The foot should stay on the ground. Roll the child towards you by pulling on the far leg. Keep the hip and knee of the upper leg at right angles. Ensure that the airway is open and check the child regularly. The child should be turned onto the opposite side after 30 minutes to rest arm that they were laying on.

Neonatal examination

The aims of the neonatal examination are:

1. Detection of uncommon but serious conditions (e.g. cyanotic congenital heart disease)
2. Detection of asymptomatic conditions (e.g. club foot)
3. Providing reassurance to parents
4. Explaining common variations
5. Allowing the parents to ask questions

'**Baby X is 10 days old. Please perform a neonatal examination.**'

Score Sheet

Scores: 1 = Not attempted; 2 = Attempted, unsatisfactory; 3 = Attempted, satisfactory

Action	1	2	3
1. Introduces self, checks identity, consent and positions appropriately			
2. Assesses gestational age, birthweight and centile			
3. Assesses muscle tone			
4. Examines head circumference and fontanelles			
5. Inspection of the face, eyes, ears, palate and neck			
6. Palpates pulses			
7. Examines the chest and auscultates the heart and lungs			
8. Examines the abdomen			
9. Asks about urine/meconium and examines the anus and genitalia			
10. Inspects the back and spine			
11. Tests for developmental dysplasia of the hip and looks for other skeletal deformities			
12. Tests the primitive reflexes			
13. Dresses the baby, summarizes findings and addresses any parental concerns			
Overall score		/39	

1. All clinical examinations should begin with simple checks remembered using the acronym **WIIPPE**: **W**ash hands, **I**ntroduction, **I**dentity, **P**ermission, **P**osition, **E**xposure. The neonate should be fully undressed

1. Cyanosis (peripheral cyanosis is common on the first day, traumatic cyanosis such as that caused by the umbilical cord around the neck, or presentation at birth may also cause blue discolouration of the skin)
2. Distorted head shape, eyelid swelling, subconjunctival haemorrhages (secondary to delivery)
3. Milia (caused by follicular keratin deposits particularly on the nose and cheeks)
4. Cysts (usually on the floor of the mouth or gums)
5. Epstein's pearls (along midline of palate)
6. Mongolian blue spot (bluish discolouration at the base of the spine and buttocks usually in Afro-Caribbean or Asian babies)
7. 'Stork bites' (pink macules present on the neck, upper eyelids and mid-forehead)
8. Umbilical hernia (usually occurs in Afro-Caribbean babies)
9. Positional talipes (the foot can be dorsiflexed to touch the anterior aspect of the leg unlike in talipes equinovarus)

and placed on a bed in order to observe general appearance and movements. The examination should ideally be performed with both parents present. Take this opportunity to explore any immediate concerns the parents may have. Explain that many abnormalities are minor and most of them will resolve. Common abnormalities are listed in the box above. In a neonatal examination, it is important to be opportunistic. For example, if the baby is calm it may be more appropriate to auscultate rather than when the baby becomes distressed. Therefore, the above structure should be used as a guide only.

2. Begin by measuring the gestational age, birthweight and centile. If the baby is below the tenth centile, they are considered small for dates. The baby may have suffered from intrauterine growth restriction. This may be symmetrical or asymmetrical, and this is dependent on whether the abdominal circumference is on the same or in a lower centile to that of the head. Conversely, a mother with diabetes may have had a large-for-dates baby. An average birthweight is 3.5 kg.

3. Assess muscle tone. Observe spontaneous limb movements. There is a smooth, flowing quality to the movements in normal term babies.

4. The head circumference is a rough estimate of brain size and should be approximately 35 cm. This is measured with a paper tape above the eyebrows and ears around to the occiput. Macrocephaly may be due to conditions such as hydrocephalus or chronic subdural haematomas. Microcephaly may be due to infection or intrauterine hypoxia. In a baby, the sutures and fontanelles remain open. The anterior fontanelle closes by 12–18 months. The posterior fontanelle should be closed 2–3 months after birth. A tense anterior fontanelle, when not crying, may be a sign of raised intracranial

pressure, and cranial ultrasound should be performed urgently. Premature fusion of sutures indicates cranisynostosis. Sutural overriding can be a normal phenomenon seen in the immediate neonatal period.

a. An abnormal facies, particularly in the presence of other abnormalities, may suggest a congenital syndrome. If in doubt, expert advice from a consultant paediatrician should be sought.

b. It is important to look for cyanosis. In the first few days, peripheral cyanosis is common (see the above box). However, central cyanosis should always be investigated and may be caused by cardiac or respiratory disorders (see the table below).

Respiratory	Cardiac	Other
Respiratory distress syndrome	Tetralogy of Fallot	Seizure
Infection	Transposition of the great vessels	Apnoea
Pneumothorax	Ebstein's anomaly	
Pleural effusion		

c. It is also important to look for jaundice. Jaundice in the first 24 hours is always pathological and the likely causes of jaundice change with the time course (see the table below). It is important not to miss jaundice as unconjugated bilirubin can cause neurotoxicity and can lead to death or kernicterus if the baby survives. This needs to be treated with phototherapy or exchange transfusion based on the levels of serum bilirubin.

Jaundice <24 hours	Jaundice >24 hours to 3 weeks
ABO/Rhesus incompatibility	Physiological
Spherocytosis	Breast milk
G6PD deficiency	Crigler–Najjar syndrome
Intrauterine infection, e.g. hepatitis, CMV	

d. Use an ophthalmoscope to examine the retina. Remember to check for the red reflex. If it is absent, this may be due to cataracts or a retinoblastoma and urgent referral to the ophthalmologist is required.

e. Examine the size and position of the ears and check for the presence of an auditory canal.

f. Inspect the mouth for cyanosis and carefully inspect the palate. Explain to the parents that you wish to examine the palate with a finger (ensure you wash your hands). Palpate the palate feeling for a cleft (posterior palate).

g. Thoroughly inspect the neck for thyroid cysts or enlargement as well as for swellings particularly of the sternocleidomastoid. Check for webbing of the neck (seen in Turner's syndrome). Examine the range of rotation of the head and palpate the clavicles. If a fracture is suspected, X-rays should be performed.

5. Palpate the brachial and femoral pulses. A reduction in pulse pressure between upper and lower limb pulses would suggest coarctation of the aorta. Conversely, an increase in pulse pressure suggests a patent ductus arteriosus.

6. Observe chest wall movement. The respiratory rate should be between 30 and 50 breaths per minute. It is important to remember that babies are periodic breathers and as such may not breathe for short periods of time (5–10 seconds). Expiratory grunting, head bobbing, tracheal tug and flaring of the nostrils are signs of respiratory distress. Next examine the praecordium. Begin by palpating for the apex beat. Auscultate the praecordium. A normal heart rate is between 120 and 160 beats per minute. During sleep this may drop to 80–90 beats per minute. The intensity of a murmur may not be very useful in a neonate as relatively benign lesions such as ventricular septal defects may result in loud murmurs, whereas severe structural heart disease may not produce a murmur. Auscultate the lungs both anteriorly and posteriorly.

7. Remove the nappy at this point, if you have not already done so. It may be possible to see abdominal organs and the liver edge on inspection. Observe for visible peristalsis. It is important to look for signs of bleeding and infection at the umbilicus. As opposed to umbilical hernias, inguinal hernias require a surgical opinion. Palpate the abdomen, looking for signs of distress in the baby's face. The liver usually extends up to 2 cm below the right costal margin and is palpated for from the right iliac fossa towards the right costal margin. The spleen tip may also be palpated on the opposite side. The lower pole of the left kidney may also be palpated. Ballot the kidneys by placing one hand anteriorly and one hand posteriorly while balloting upwards with the posterior hand. Any other masses felt require further investigation. If the abdomen is distended, one must consider gaseous distention, fluid or enlarged organs. An abdominal X-ray (AXR) is indicated followed by an abdominal ultrasound if no obvious cause is found. Auscultation is performed by placing the stethoscope below and to the right of the umbilicus. One should listen for 1 minute before deciding bowel sounds are not present. This may suggest obstruction and should be investigated as described above.

8. Ask the parents if the baby has passed urine and meconium. In males, the scrotum should be palpated to ensure that the testes have descended. Ensure that they are of similar size and do not appear blue as this may be a sign of testicular torsion. Examine for hypospadias where the urethral opening may be in a more proximal location on the ventral aspect of the penis. In females, the clitoris may be prominent, but clitoromegaly may also be a sign of masculinization. Examine the anus for patency.

9. Inspect the back and palpate the spine. Midline dimples or hair may suggest a neural tube defect.

10. Examine the hips to assess for developmental dysplasia of the hip. It is best to perform this at the end as this is the most uncomfortable

1. Barlow's test: tests for a hip joint that is reduced but dislocatable
- Stabilize the pelvis by gripping the sacrum and pubic symphysis with one hand
- Use the other hand to provide backwards pressure on the greater trochanter
- A clunk is felt if the femoral head subluxes
- Pressure in the opposite direction should return the femoral head to its normal position

2. Ortolani's test: tests for a hip joint that is dislocated but reducible
- Place the baby on its back with its knees and hips flexed to 90°
- Place your thumbs on either side of the baby's knee with an index finger over the greater trochanter
- Abduct the hips through 90°
- A clunk is felt if the femoral head relocates back into the acetabulum

examination for the baby. The two main tests – Barlow's test and Ortolani's test – are outlined in the boxes above. If either test is positive, an orthopaedic referral is required.

Ensure that you have counted the number digits on both the toes and fingers. Check for deformities. If the baby cannot dorsiflex and externally rotate the foot, a diagnosis of club foot can be made. A calcaneus deformity can be diagnosed if the foot cannot be plantarflexed to 45° beyond a right angle. These conditions require an orthopaedic referral.

11. Check for primitive reflexes such as the palmar grasp reflex, rooting reflex and the Moro reflex.
    a. Palmar grasp reflex
        Place both index fingers in the neonate's palms to elicit the palmar grasp reflex.
    b. Rooting reflex
        The baby turns its head and opens its mouth in response to touching the lateral aspect of its upper lip. May not be present if the baby has just had a large feed.
    c. Moro reflex
        This is performed by placing an arm under the baby's shoulders, releasing the head and catching it again. This causes bilateral extension followed by flexion of the arms.
12. The baby should be dressed and handed back to the parents. Take the time to explain the examination findings and their implications, and answer any questions the parents may have.

I examined Baby X who was born 10 days ago. On inspection, he was comfortable at rest. His birthweight, head circumference and centile on the growth charts suggested that he was of normal size. He was pink, warm and well-perfused. He was neither cyanosed nor jaundiced, and his tone was normal. Cardiovascular and respiratory examinations were normal. However, on abdominal examination, I noted an umbilical hernia. Bowel sounds were normal. Orthopaedic examination demonstrated a positive Ortolani's test, but examination of the spine was unremarkable. Primitive reflexes were present and normal.

These findings would be most consistent with a diagnosis of a baby with an umbilical hernia and possible developmental dysplasia of the hip. To complete my examination, I would like to refer this baby to orthopaedics.

Developmental examination

'You meet your first outpatient as an FY2 in general paediatrics, a young boy who attends with his mother. Please perform a developmental examination. You are allowed to ask the mother questions.'

Score Sheet

Scores: 1 = Not attempted; 2 = Attempted, unsatisfactory; 3 = Attempted, satisfactory

Action	1	2	3
1. Introduces self, checks child's name and date of birth, and establishes rapport			
2. Assesses gross motor function			
3. Assesses vision and fine motor function			
4. Assesses hearing, speech and language			
5. Assesses social and emotional behaviour			
6. Summarizes findings and gives a development age for each broad category assessed			
Overall score		/18	

1. Introduce yourself, check the child's details (name and date of birth) and confirm the relationship of any attending adults.
2. Child development should be considered within four broad categories: gross motor; vision and fine motor; hearing, speech and language; social, emotional and behavioural. In order to assess for development, it is necessary to know about the major developmental milestones (below).

The developmental history is essential to elicit in addition to a formal developmental assessment. This provides valuable information regarding whether a child has reached his or her milestones. In the developmental assessment itself, it is important to observe the child throughout the consultation as this can provide important social, emotional and behavioural information.

3. **Gross motor**

   Newborn: Posture is symmetrical. The infant shows head lag on being pulled up, by the wrists, from lying to sitting.

   6–8 weeks: Able to raise head to 45°.

   12 weeks: Head control achieved.

   6–8 months: Able to sit without support (rounded back at 6 months and straight back at 8 months).

   8–9 months: Begins to crawl.

   10 months: Uses furniture to walk around (cruising).

   12 months: Unsteady gait, broad based.

   15 months: Able to walk alone.

   The general approach is to take a best guess at the age, and aim to do an appropriate activity, then adjust if required. For example, if you think the child is around 8 months, see if he or she is able to crawl (you can ask for the parent's help). If the child is able, then see if he or she can cruise. If the child is unable to crawl, see if he or she can sit without support. The same principle can be applied to the other categories.

4. **Vision and fine motor**

   Simple equipment is required for the remainder of the assessment and may include crayons and paper, cubes, a picture book, miniature toys such as a tea set and balls. Allowing the child to play with the toys gives the assessor an idea as to the stage of development.

   Newborn: Only able to follow a face in the midline.

   6 weeks: Turns the head to follow a moving object.

   4 months: Reaches for toys.

   6 months: Able to transfers toys between hands.

   9 months: Develops pincer grip.

   16–18 months: Uses a crayon to make marks.

   14 months to 4 years: 18 months: able to build a tower of three blocks; 2 years: able to build a tower of six blocks; 2.5 years: able to build a tower of eight blocks or a train with four blocks; 3 years: able to build a bridge (from a model); and 4 years: able to build steps (having been shown).

   2–5 years: 2 years: able to draw a line; 3 years: able to draw a circle; 4 years: able to draw a cross; 4.5 years: able to draw a square; and >5 years: able to draw a triangle. The child is usually able to copy these shapes 6 months earlier than being able to draw them.

5. **Hearing, speech and language**

   Remember you are allowed to ask the parent questions as there may be some things you are unable to elicit during the examination, such as the ability of the child to use simple phrases.

   Newborn: Startles upon hearing loud noises.

   3–4 months: Begins to vocalize with sounds.

   7 months: Responds to sounds out of sight by turning the head.

   7–10 months: At 7 months sounds are used indiscriminately, but by 10 months sounds are used discriminately, e.g. mama, dada.

12 months: Has 2–3 words other than mama and dada.
18 months: Has 6–10 words and can show parts of the body.
20–24 months: Able to use words to create simple phrases.
2½ to 3 years: Talks in 3–4 word sentences.

6. **Social, emotional and behavioural**
   6 weeks: Exhibits social smiling.
   6–8 months: Able to put food in their mouth.
   10–12 months: Can wave goodbye.
   12 months: Uses two hands to drink from a cup.
   18 months: Able to use a spoon to feed.
   18–24 months: Exhibits symbolic play.
   2 years: Is dry during the day.
   3 years: Is interactive play.
7. Summarize your findings by giving an age range (you are not expected to give an exact age) for each of the broad areas of development you have assessed. For example, 'He is able to cruise holding onto furniture, but cannot yet crawl, so his gross motor age is around 8–10 months'. You can then give your overall assessment of the child's developmental age (again you can give a range).

Cardiovascular examination

'Martha is 11 years old. She has been recently diagnosed with Turner's syndrome. Please perform a cardiovascular examination.'

Score Sheet

Scores: 1 = Not attempted; 2 = Attempted, unsatisfactory; 3 = Attempted, satisfactory

Action	1	2	3
Introduction			
1. Performs introduction, washes hands and exposes patient			
Inspection and peripheral examination			
2. Gross observation of child and surroundings			
3. Elicits respiratory rate			
4. Examines the hands			
5. Examines the pulse, blood pressure (mentions)			
6. Inspects the jugular venous pressure (JVP)			
7. Inspects the face, eyes, mouth and teeth			
8. Inspects the chest			
Palpation			
9. Palpates the apex			
10. Palpates for heaves/thrills			

Continued

Action	1	2	3
Auscultation			
11. Auscultates the heart			
12. Auscultates the lung bases			
Other examination			
13. Offers to check for sacral/peripheral oedema, hepatomegaly and peripheral pulses			
Summary			
14. Summarizes findings and suggests further investigations			
Overall score		/42	

1. All clinical examinations should begin with simple checks remembered using the acronym **WIIPPE: W**ash hands, **I**ntroduction, **I**dentity, **P**ermission, **P**osition, **E**xposure. Ideally the child should be positioned at 45° with their chest fully exposed.

2. Begin by observing the child and his or her surroundings. There may be clues around the bedside including ECG monitoring, oxygen (note the oxygen delivery method, e.g. nasal cannulae, face mask, venturi mask, non-rebreather mask), medications and infusions.

   Note the colour of the child. Do they appear cyanosed, tachypnoeic and, particularly in the case of younger children, lethargic or irritable?

3. It may be useful at this point to record the child's respiratory rate. This varies with the age of the child (see the table below).

Age	Breaths per minute
Neonate	30–50
2–5 years	24–30
5–12 years	20–24
<12 years	12–20

4. Examine the hands for:
   a. **Clubbing:** This is defined as an increase in the nail and nail bed angle, increased fluctuation of the nail bed and increased curvature of the nail. Cardiovascular causes of clubbing are:
      i. Infective endocarditis (subacute)
      ii. Congenital cyanotic heart disease
      iii. Atrial myxoma
   b. **Peripheral cyanosis:** The child may be peripherally cyanosed (noted in the hands and feet, sometimes in the lips, but not in the tongue). This is either due to cold, poor circulation or severe central cyanosis. The capillary refill time can be used to test circulation and should be less than 3 seconds. This is performed by pressing down on the pulp of the finger for 5 seconds and recording the time taken

for the finger to turn from white to pink. Cyanosis is defined as a concentration of deoxygenated haemoglobin of >50 g/L. Central cyanosis is evidenced by blue discolouration of the lips and tongue. In patients with a normal haemoglobin, one would expect cyanosis at oxygen saturations of below 90% (PaO_2 8KPa). N.B. In patients with polycythaemia, cyanosis occurs with a higher PO_2, and conversely in anaemic patients, cyanosis may not become apparent until the patient is severely hypoxic as the necessary levels of deoxygenated haemoglobin will not be reached prior to this point. Note that in babies it is difficult to assess for cyanosis, and so an ear probe can be employed to measure saturations, if available.

5. Examine the wrists and arms for:

a. **Pulse:** In younger children (up to toddler age), the pulse is best felt brachially. In older children and adults, the radial pulse is traditionally used. If the brachial pulse is absent, a previous operation such as repair of coarctation of the aorta may have been performed. Record the heart rate. The heart rate varies with age (see the table below) and emotional state of the child. If it is irregular, determine if this is regularly irregular or irregularly irregular. N.B. As there can be variations in stroke volume, using the radial artery to determine irregularity may not be accurate. Using your stethoscope to listen at the apex of the heart should clarify the situation.

Age (years)	Beats per minute
<1	110–160
2–5	95–140
5–12	80–120
>12	60–100

b. **Radio-femoral delay:** Palpate the radial and femoral pulse at the same time. The femoral pulse is best measured at the mid-inguinal point, midway between the pubic symphysis and the anterior superior iliac spine. This is useful in young patients to determine whether they may have an underlying diagnosis of coarctation of the aorta. If this is positive, look for other signs suggestive of coarctation including: collateral vessel bruits heard around the scapula, systolic murmur and upper limb hypertension in comparison to the lower limbs. Allow for a 10 mmHg discrepancy between blood pressures in the arms and a 20 mmHg increase in blood pressure between the arms and the legs.

c. **Collapsing pulse:** Hold your fingers flat across the radial pulse. Ask the child if they have any pain in their shoulder. Lift the forearm above the head. If the pulse is collapsing (suggestive of aortic regurgitation), you should feel a forceful impulse throughout the forearm. This is not always easy to ascertain in younger children.

d. **Blood pressure:** Measure the blood pressure (in the exam, just mention that you would do this, and only perform if asked). It is important to use the correct cuff size. The cuff should completely encircle the bicep and cover two-thirds of the length of the arm. It is important to put a child at ease. One way to do this is to practice on a toy or parent to demonstrate that there is nothing to worry about. In the very young, it may be difficult to auscultate for a blood pressure, and in this case, palpation of the brachial pulse may be performed. The reading can then be compared to centile charts for blood pressure. Pulse pressure is the difference between the systolic and diastolic blood pressures. This is characteristically narrow in aortic stenosis and wide in aortic regurgitation. If the child is complaining of postural symptoms, it is appropriate to perform a postural blood pressure measurement. The blood pressure is recorded with the child lying down and within 1 minute of standing up. A systolic drop of 20 mmHg or a 10 mmHg diastolic drop is significant.

6. Inspect the JVP

The JVP may be examined in older children as in adults. Ask the child to turn the head to the left side. If the head is turned too far over, the sternocleidomastoid becomes prominent and the JVP becomes difficult to see. In these cases, it may be easier to see the JVP with the neck extended backwards. The JVP can be seen along the line of the internal jugular vein along the border of the sternocleidomastoid (from between the two heads of the sternocleidomastoid to the earlobe). The JVP can be distinguished from the carotid pulse as illustrated in the box below. If the JVP is low, it may not be seen, and if it is high, it may be flickering at the earlobe. The JVP is measured from the sternal angle vertically upwards and can be up to 4 cm. The JVP waveform has several characteristics. The A wave is seen in atrial contraction and may be absent in atrial fibrillation. Giant A waves, or cannon A waves, can be seen in complete heart block; V waves are caused by ventricular systole against a closed valve. If this is prominent, there is likely to be tricuspid regurgitation. If the JVP is elevated, this may be a sign of heart failure, pulmonary hypertension or superior

CHARACTERISTICS OF JVP
1. Bifid.
2. Impalpable.
3. Varies with respiration (falls on inspiration) and position.
4. Increases transiently with pressure on the abdomen. This is performed by asking the child if they have any pain in their abdomen and then applying pressure to the upper abdomen for 20 seconds. If the JVP remains persistently elevated for this time, this is a positive abdomino-jugular reflux sign.

vena cava obstruction. If the JVP rises on inspiration, this is Kussmaul's sign and suggests constrictive pericarditis or cardiac tamponade.

Palpate the carotid pulse: Unlike the radial pulse, one can use the carotid pulse to comment on the character and volume of the pulse. A small-volume, slow-rising pulse is characteristic of aortic stenosis.

7. Examine the face, eyes, mouth and teeth
   a. Examine the face for syndromic facies which may point you in the direction of congenital heart disease.
   b. On examination of the eyes, conjunctival pallor suggests anaemia. On fundoscopy, Roth spots may be seen. These are flame-shaped retinal haemorrhages often found in infective endocarditis.
   c. Inspect the mouth for signs of central cyanosis and plethoric facies caused by polycythaemia in cyanotic heart disease. Bluish discolouration of the tongue and mucous membranes suggests central cyanosis. This is best seen by asking the child to lift his or her tongue to the roof of the mouth.
   d. Examine the teeth as caries may be a risk factor for infective endocarditis. Examine for the high arched palate of Marfan's syndrome and petechiae suggestive of infective endocarditis.
8. Examine the chest for scars. Sternotomy or thoracotomy scars might suggest repair of congenital heart defects such as closure of a patent ductus arteriosus or repair of coarctation of the aorta. Pacemaker scars may be visible, and there may also be current or healed drain or vascular access sites. Note the age of the scars and if they appear healthy. A precordial bulge suggests enlargement of the heart and a ventricular impulse may also be visible suggesting left ventricular hypertrophy.
9. Palpate for the apex beat. The apex beat should be felt in the fourth (<7 years old) or fifth intercostal space (ICS) (>7 years old) in the midclavicular line. This may not be palpable in 40% of people, particularly obese children or those with hyperinflation. Ventricular dilatation causes a displaced apex beat. Dextrocardia is diagnosed if the apex beat is palpable on the right side. It can be difficult to determine the character of the apex beat. The easiest way to subdivide the nature of the apex beat is to classify it into normal, volume overloaded, pressure overloaded or a combination. In volume overload, the apex beat is diffuse and displaced such as in mitral or aortic regurgitation, ischaemic heart disease leading to damage to the ventricles or dilated cardiomyopathy. In pressure overload, the apex beat is forceful such as in aortic stenosis or hypertension. A tapping apex beat occurs in mitral stenosis (palpable first sound), and a double impulse is suggestive of hypertrophic cardiomyopathy.
10. Using the heel of your hand, palpate for heaves. Place your hand over the left sternal edge to feel for a right ventricular heave. This produces a sensation of the hand rising off the chest in time with the cardiac impulse. Thrills should be palpated with the fingertips in the mitral region (the apex), the tricuspid region (lower left sternal edge, fourth ICS), the aortic region

(upper right sternal edge, second ICS) and the pulmonary region (upper left sternal edge, second ICS). A thrill is a palpable murmur and gives the sensation of a vibration or buzzing beneath the fingers. Parasternal thrills are due to a ventricular septal defect.

11. When auscultating, time the heart sounds with the carotid pulse. Use the diaphragm to listen over the mitral, tricuspid, pulmonary and aortic regions. This is best to listen to high-pitched sounds. Repeat using the bell of the stethoscope in order to detect low-pitched sounds.

    a. **Heart sounds:** The first and second heart sounds (S1 and S2) are caused by closure of the heart valves, the mitral/tricuspid and aortic/pulmonary valves, respectively. A loud S2 is caused by pulmonary hypertension. Splitting of S2 (separate sounds for aortic and pulmonary valve closures) can occur during inspiration, and a variable time gap between the S2 sounds can be normal. If there is fixed splitting, the child is likely to have an atrial septal defect. A third heart sound, S3, can be normal in young patients through passive filling of the ventricles but may be suggestive of heart failure. Causes include rapid ventricular filling (mitral regurgitation, ventricular septal defect) or poor left ventricular function (e.g. dilated cardiomyopathy). A fourth heart sound, S4, is caused by atrial contraction against a ventricle that is non-compliant and is pathological. Causes include ventricular hypertrophy, e.g. from aortic stenosis or hypertrophic cardiomyopathy.

    b. **Murmurs** should be characterized as follows:

       i. **Timing:** systolic/diastolic
       ii. **Duration:** e.g. ejection systolic, pansystolic, early diastolic
       iii. **Volume:** 1–2 difficult to hear; 3, easily audible, no thrill; 4–6, loud with thrill
       iv. **Site of maximum intensity:** e.g. mitral, tricuspid, pulmonary, aortic
       v. **Radiation:** e.g. carotids, axilla, back

    Radiation can be detected by listening around into the axilla or into the neck. Other sounds that might be heard are a pericardial rub which sounds like footsteps crunching fresh snow.

    Manoeuvres can be used, as in adults, to increase the intensity of the murmur and therefore make it easier to characterize. Right-sided murmurs are heard best on inspiration. Left-sided murmurs are heard best on expiration. This can be remembered by the acronym RILE (right inspiration, left expiration). The two most common manoeuvres are turning the child onto their left side and asking them to take a breath in and out, and hold it at the end of expiration. Use the bell to auscultate the apex listening for mitral stenosis. In order to detect aortic regurgitation, listen with the diaphragm at the lower left sternal edge with the child leaning forward. Ask the child to take a breath in and out and hold it at the end of expiration. In children, it is also important to listen between the scapulae and over any possible vascular swellings such as over the thyroid gland or limbs.

12. Ask the child to sit forward and listen for crackles in the lung bases suggestive of oedema.
13. Further examinations can be offered, and performed at the examiner's request.
    a. **Sacral oedema:** Ask the child if he or she has any pain in his or her lower back and feel the sacrum for sacral oedema. Press firmly on the sacrum for 15 seconds. If an indentation of your finger is left behind, there is pitting oedema. This also provides an opportunity to listen between the scapulae for radiation of a murmur.
    b. **Pulsatile hepatomegaly:** Lie the child flat and examine the liver (see Abdominal examination section). A liver edge of 1–2 cm below the costal margin is normal, but the liver may be enlarged and pulsatile in tricuspid regurgitation. Tender hepatomegaly is indicative of cardiac failure.
    c. **Peripheral oedema:** Check the ankles for pitting oedema in a similar fashion to that noted earlier. Remember to see how far up the legs the pitting oedema is present as in severe cases this can be as far up as the abdomen.
    d. **Peripheral pulses:** Palpate for the dorsalis pedis and posterior tibial pulses.
    e. **Growth charts:** It is also important to plot the height and weight of the child on a centile chart to see if these measurements are appropriate for his or her age.
14. Thank the parents and, if appropriate, the child. Provide a summary of your examination findings and suggest further investigations. For example:

> *I examined Martha, who is 11 years old and has a recent diagnosis of Turner's syndrome. On general examination, she was comfortable at rest with no peripheral stigmata of infective endocarditis. There was a slight radio-femoral delay on palpation. On examination of the precordium, the apex beat was forceful and not displaced. I heard an ejection systolic murmur which was best heard at the back. Her chest was clear, and there was no peripheral oedema. Abdominal examination was unremarkable, and pedal pulses were palpable bilaterally.*
>
> *These findings would be consistent with a diagnosis of coarctation of the aorta.*
>
> *To complete my examination I would like to perform bilateral blood pressures as well as blood pressures in the arms and the legs. I would also like to record the oxygen saturations, perform an ECG and order a CXR.*

Questions

1. What are the features of an innocent murmur?
   The box below summarizes features of an innocent murmur and gives examples of murmurs that are not concerning. However, if unsure, expert advice should always be sought.

Clinical findings:
Asymptomatic, no other findings
No diastolic component
No thrills
No radiation
Remember the S's: short, soft, systolic, small (no radiation)

Normal murmurs:
Pulmonary murmur: systolic murmur best heard in the second intercostal space.
Still's murmur: short murmur best heard with the child supine in the fourth ICS.

2. Give some examples of heart murmurs you may find in a child.
   The characteristics of more common heart murmurs are found in the table below:

Diagnosis	Location of the murmur	Character of the murmur
Acyanotic heart disease		
Aortic stenosis	Aortic area radiating to carotids	Ejection systolic
Coarctation of the aorta	Back	Systolic
Pulmonary stenosis	Pulmonary area	Ejection systolic
Atrial septal defect	Upper left sternal edge	Ejection systolic
Ventricular septal defect	Lower left sternal edge	Pansystolic
Patent ductus arteriosus	Left clavicle	Continuous murmur
Cyanotic heart disease		
Tetralogy of Fallot	Left sternal edge	Ejection systolic
Transposition of the great vessels	Usually no murmur but may be a systolic murmur from increased flow in the left ventricular outflow tract (pulmonary tract)	

3. What further investigations may be appropriate to perform following a cardiovascular examination?
   Investigations to complete the examination will depend on the underlying diagnosis obtained from a thorough history and examination and can be broken down in the following manner:
   a. Immediate bedside tests
      i. O_2 saturations
      ii. ECG
      iii. Fundoscopy
      iv. Urine dipstick (for microscopic haematuria)
   b. Laboratory tests
      i. Blood tests
      ii. Blood cultures (if infective endocarditis is suspected)

c. Imaging
   i. CXR
   ii. Echocardiogram
   iii. CT/MRI
d. Invasive tests/outpatient tests
   i. Exercise tests/stress echocardiogram
   ii. Angiography

Abdominal examination

'Harry is 4 years old. He has been complaining about a lump in his abdomen. Please perform an abdominal examination.'

Score Sheet

Scores: 1 = Not attempted; 2 = Attempted, unsatisfactory; 3 = Attempted, satisfactory

Action	1	2	3
Introduction			
1. Performs introduction, washes hands and exposes patient			
Inspection and peripheral examination			
2. Gross observation of child and surroundings			
3. Examines the hands			
4. Checks the pulse			
5. Examines for cervical lymphadenopathy			
6. Inspects the face, eyes, mouth and teeth			
7. Inspects the abdomen			
Palpation			
8. Palpates for abdominal tenderness			
9. Palpates the liver, spleen and kidneys			
Percussion			
10. Percusses for the liver, spleen (and any masses if appropriate)			
11. Percusses for ascites (if relevant)			
Auscultation			
12. Auscultates for bowel sounds			
Other examination			
13. Offers to perform genital examination (in boys) or rectal examination (in infants)			
Summary			
14. Summarizes findings and suggests further investigations			
Overall score		/42	

1. All clinical examinations should begin with simple checks remembered using the acronym **WIIPPE: W**ash hands, **I**ntroduction, **I**dentity, **P**ermission, **P**osition, **E**xposure. Ideally the child should be positioned flat and exposed from the nipple to the pubis symphysis.
2. Begin by observing the child and his or her surroundings. There may be clues around the bedside including intravenous infusions, NG tubes, medications including supplements, as well as monitoring equipment.

   Note the colour of the child. Does the child appear jaundiced and, particularly in the case of younger children, lethargic or irritable? Once the child is exposed, one can assess his or her nutritional status. In malabsorption states secondary to coeliac disease or malnutrition for example, the child may have wasted buttocks and cachectic limbs.
3. Examine the hands for:
   a. **Clubbing:** This is defined as an increase in the nail–nail bed angle, increased fluctuation of the nail bed and increased curvature of the nail. Common gastrointestinal causes of clubbing are:
      i. Crohn's disease
      ii. Ulcerative colitis
      iii. Cirrhosis
   b. **Capillary refill:** The capillary refill time can be used to test circulation and should be less than 3 seconds. This is performed by pressing down on the pulp of the finger for 5 seconds and recording the time taken for the finger to turn from white to pink.
   c. **Palmar erythema:** Turn the hands over to look for palmar erythema. This is suggestive of liver disease.

      Inspect the skin for signs of liver disease such as jaundice or spider naevi. Spider naevi are caused by hyperoestrogenaemia. They are commonly seen on the upper torso in the distribution of the superior vena cava. Up to five spider naevi may be normal. They consist of a central arteriole surrounded by small veins carrying the blood away. They can be characterized by pressing down on the spider naevi. When released, the spider naevi will refill from the centre outwards.
4. Check the pulse. In younger children (up to toddler age), the pulse is best felt brachially. Record the heart rate. The heart rate varies with age (see the table below) and emotional state of the child.

Age (years)	Beats per minute
<1	110–160
2–5	95–140
5–12	80–120
>12	60–100

5. Palpate for lymphadenopathy. This is best carried out from behind the child, asking him or her to rest his or her chin on your hands. This may be performed when examining the back of the chest to reduce the number of

times the child has to sit forward and back. There is no hard and fast rule for the order of examination but a systematic approach ensures that all lymph node groups are examined. Lymph node groups to cover include submental, mandibular, preauricular, postauricular, anterior cervical chain, posterior cervical chain and occipital lymph nodes. Enlargement of lymph nodes is commonly due to infection but malignancy should be considered. One should examine the axillary and inguinal lymph nodes if lymphadenopathy is detected.

6. Examine the eyes for any evidence of anaemia (conjunctival pallor) or scleral icterus. The latter is best seen by pulling the upper eyelid upwards and asking the child to look downwards.

   Look inside the mouth and note the presence of ulcers which may be caused by inflammatory bowel disease such as Crohn's disease. Poor dentition may also be a cause of poor nutritional status and is important to note. Observe the tongue and whether it is coated.

7. Inspect the abdomen while kneeling by the child. Look for surgical scars or drain sites, noting the age of the scars and if they appear healthy. It may be possible to observe visible peristalsis suggestive of pyloric stenosis in a neonate or obstruction in an older child, or abdominal distention.

   If the distention is predominantly of the upper abdomen, the possible differentials include enlargement of the stomach secondary to pyloric stenosis or hepatomegaly and/or splenomegaly. In the lower abdomen, possibilities include masses such as a Wilm's tumour or a distended bladder. Other diagnoses to consider include significant lordosis or muscle hypotonia. Conversely, a depressed abdomen may suggest a high intestinal obstruction or dehydration. It is possible to narrow the differential further, following palpation and auscultation.

   Other points to note on inspection include abdominal movement. In older children and adults, the abdomen moves inwards on inspiration. However, in children below school age, this is described as 'abdominal breathing'. The abdomen moves outwards during inspiration. If the abdomen is peritonitic, it will not move with respiration at all. One can examine at this point for herniae or wait until the end of the examination. Divarication of the rectae seen on asking the child to lift his or her head off the bed is common, and the child and parents should be reassured. Umbilical hernias presenting at birth commonly do not pose any problems and resolve within a year. In general, inguinal hernias are best examined and become more apparent when the child is standing. These are more common in males. Hernias should be palpated and the cough impulse tested if the child is able to do so. It is also important to see whether the hernia is reducible. The hernia should be auscultated for bowel sounds if bowel content is suspected. Inguinal hernias generally require surgery, and a referral should be made promptly or urgently if there are any signs of intestinal obstruction. Prominent blood vessels may be apparent in portal hypertension secondary to liver disease around the umbilicus (caput medusae). Distended blood vessels may also occur in a child fed by parenteral nutrition requiring central venous access.

8. It is important to ensure that the child is relaxed before palpating the abdomen. It may be appropriate to reposition the child, for example onto the mother's lap. Ask the child if he or she has any pain anywhere. Palpate the nine quadrants of the abdomen starting on the opposite side to the pain, first superficially and then more deeply. Watch the child's face for any signs of distress. Feel for tenderness, voluntary and involuntary guarding, masses and muscle tone. Guarding may not be elicited on palpation, and there are other signs of peritoneal irritation. For example, the child may have increased pain on coughing and moving.

   If a child is reluctant to allow you to palpate their abdomen, use his or her hand to palpate the abdomen or put your hand on top of the child's hand. Rebound tenderness, assessing for peritonitis, should not be performed; the same information can be elicited if the child has percussion tenderness. If appendicitis is suspected, the psoas muscle test can be performed. This involves flexing the right hip and applying downwards pressure. If this elicits pain there is peritoneal irritation. If the child complains of pain but there is not thought to be any, distraction techniques can be employed such as asking the child about his or her school day or toys.

9. Palpate for the following:

   a. **Liver:** The liver should be palpated from the right iliac fossa to the right costal margin. If the child is old enough, ask him or her to breathe in as you palpate. Move upwards by 1 cm each time until you reach the costal margin. It is normal for the liver to extend up 1–2 cm below the right costal margin in infants and young children. This is measured in the mid-clavicular line. The liver moves with respiration and one cannot get above it.

   b. **Spleen:** The spleen should be palpated from the right iliac fossa diagonally towards the left costal margin. If the child is old enough, ask him or her to breathe in as you palpate. Move diagonally by 1 cm each time until you reach the costal margin. The spleen moves with respiration, and one cannot get above it. There may be a notch if the spleen is enlarged. In infants, the spleen may be felt 1–2 cm below the costal margin in the mid-clavicular line. If one is uncertain whether the spleen is palpable, the child can be turned onto his or her right side and the spleen should be palpated using a bimanual approach.

   c. **Kidneys:** In children, the kidneys should not be palpable except for in the newborn. Ballot the kidneys by placing one hand anteriorly and one hand posteriorly while balloting upwards with the posterior hand. If palpable, the kidneys should move with respiration and it should be possible to get above them. Enlargement unilaterally may be due to Wilms' tumour, renal vein thrombosis or bilaterally due to polycystic kidney disease or bilateral obstructive disease. Any masses should be characterized by site, size, shape, surface, edge, consistency, fluctuance, mobility, tenderness and temperature. Any masses felt should also be percussed to elucidate possible components, as well as auscultated for bruits and bowel sounds.

10. One should percuss for the liver and spleen as well as any masses. Depending on whether you are right-handed or left-handed, percussion is performed differently. A right-handed technique will be discussed here. To percuss the liver, start in the right iliac fossa and move upwards towards the costal margin. Similarly, to percuss the spleen, start in the right iliac fossa and move diagonally towards the left costal margin. Place your left hand flat on the abdomen with the fingers separated. Press the middle finger down into the abdomen gently and raise the other fingers off the abdomen. Strike the middle finger with the tip of the right middle finger using a swinging movement from the wrist. As with palpation, move by 1 cm and repeat. The liver and spleen are both dull to percussion. Perform the same technique for any masses felt.

11. If the abdomen is diffusely distended, ascites remains a possible diagnosis. The test for ascites is shifting dullness. Percuss outwards from the umbilicus to the right side. Keep your finger at the point where the percussion note becomes dull. Roll the child onto their left side and wait for 30 seconds. Percuss over your finger to see whether the dull percussion note has now become resonant. This is suggestive of ascites. Eliciting a fluid thrill is an alternative test for ascites. Ask an assistant to place their hand along the midline of the child's abdomen. Flick on side of the abdomen and feel for a thrill on the opposite side. This test may be falsely positive if the child is overweight.

12. Auscultate for bowel sounds below and to the right of the umbilicus. One must wait at least 30 seconds before concluding that bowel sounds are absent. Reduced bowel sounds are suggestive of ileus or peritonitis. High-pitched tinkling bowel sounds may indicate intestinal obstruction or diarrhoea. In addition, auscultate for renal artery bruits, above and to the right and left of the umbilicus, as well as over any masses.

13. In general, a rectal examination is not indicated except for in newborns to check that the anus is not imperforate. In the acute abdomen, the argument is that due to the thin abdominal wall in a young child, tenderness is easily elicited and masses are generally palpable. Some surgeons perform a rectal examination to identify a retrocaecal appendix or to identify intussusception. In the latter case, one would expect to feel a mass and stool which look like redcurrant jelly. In any case, do not attempt to perform this in the examination setting.

A genital examination should always be performed in young children but only if indicated in older children. This is particularly important in young males. One must note if the penis is of a normal size, if the testes are palpable within the scrotum and whether there are any other scrotal swellings.

It is also important to plot the height and weight of the child on a centile chart to see if these measurements are appropriate for his or her age.

14. Thank the parents and, if appropriate, the child. Provide a summary of your examination findings and suggest further investigations. For example:

I examined Harry, who is 4 years old and has been complaining about an abdominal mass. On general examination, he was comfortable at rest. He appeared cachectic with pale conjunctiva. On inspection of the abdomen, there was a non-tender mass in the right lumbar region. This was approximately 10 cm by 5 cm with a smooth surface and irregular border. It was dull to percussion, and no bowel sounds were heard.

These findings would be consistent with a diagnosis of an abdominal mass and possibly a Wilm's tumour.

To complete my examination, I would like to observe the fluid balance, perform a urine dipstick and an abdominal USS.

Questions

1. Can you name some causes of acute and chronic abdominal pain in a child?
   Possible causes of abdominal tenderness in the child include:
   a. Acute
      i. Appendicitis
      ii. Pancreatitis
      iii. Intestinal obstruction
      iv. Urinary tract infection
      v. Testicular torsion
   b. Chronic
      i. Constipation
      ii. Irritable bowel syndrome
      iii. Colic
      iv. Inflammatory bowel disease
      v. Non-specific abdominal pain of childhood

2. What are the causes of a distended abdomen?
   The possible diagnoses of a distended abdomen can be remembered by the '5 F's'.
   Faeces (constipation)
   Fat

Fluid (most likely secondary to nephrotic syndrome
Flatus (intestinal obstruction/malabsorption)
Fetus (only in post-pubescence)

3. Name some causes of hepatomegaly and splenomegaly.

Hepatomegaly
Infection: Epstein–Barr virus, hepatitis, malaria, congenital, parasites
Cardiovascular: heart failure
Liver disease: portal hypertension, polycystic kidney disease, hepatitis
Haematological: thalassaemia, sickle cell anaemia
Malignancy: leukaemia, lymphoma, Wilm's tumour, primary hepatic tumour
Metabolic: glycogen/lipid storage pathology
The liver can appear enlarged secondary to chest hyper-expansion.

Splenomegaly
Infection: malaria, leishmaniasis, infective endocarditis, viral, bacterial, parasites
Malignancy: leukaemia, lymphoma
Haematological: haemolytic anaemia

---

4. What further investigations may be appropriate to perform following an abdominal examination?
   Investigations to complete the examination will depend on the underlying diagnosis obtained from a thorough history and examination, and can be broken down in the following manner:
   a. Immediate bedside tests
      i. O_2 saturations
      ii. Fluid balance charts
      iii. Stool charts
      iv. ECG
      v. Urine dipstick (leucocytes, nitrites, glucose, haematuria, protein)
   b. Laboratory tests
      i. Blood tests (including amylase if indicated)
      ii. Blood cultures (if a septic process is suspected)
   c. Imaging
      i. AXR
      ii. USS
      iii. CT
   d. Invasive tests/outpatient tests
      i. Proctoscopy/sigmoidoscopy/colonoscopy
      ii. OGD

Respiratory examination

'Amelie is 5 years old. She has had a cough productive of sputum for the last few months. Please perform a respiratory examination.'

Score Sheet

Scores: 1 = Not attempted; 2 = Attempted, unsatisfactory; 3 = Attempted, satisfactory

Action	1	2	3
Introduction			
1. Performs introduction, washes hands and exposes patient			
Inspection and peripheral examination			
2. Gross observation of child and surroundings			
3. Measures the respiratory rate			
4. Examines the hands			
5. Checks the pulse and offers to check blood pressure			
6. Examines the neck (JVP, lymphadenopathy, trachea)			
7. Inspects face for anaemia and cyanosis			
8. Inspects the chest			
Palpation			
9. Palpates for chest expansion			
10. Palpates the apex beat			
Percussion			
11. Percusses the lung fields			
Auscultation			
12. Auscultates the lung fields			
13. Auscultates for vocal resonance			
Other examination			
14. Offers to assess peak flow			
Summary			
15. Summarizes findings and suggests further investigations			
Overall score		/45	

1. All clinical examinations should begin with simple checks remembered using the acronym **WIIPPE: W**ash hands, **I**ntroduction, **I**dentity, **P**ermission, **P**osition, **E**xposure. Ideally the child should be positioned at 45° with their chest fully exposed.
2. Begin by observing the child and his or her surroundings. Clues around the bedside include sputum pots, inhalers, oxygen (note the oxygen delivery method, e.g. nasal cannulae, face mask, venturi mask, non-rebreather mask), peak flow meter, drains and monitoring.

    The first thing to observe is whether the child looks well or unwell. Note the colour of the child. Does he or she appear cyanosed and, particularly in the case of younger children, lethargic or irritable? Look for signs of respiratory distress. Due to the flexibility of the cartilage in children, they may show sternal, intercostal and subcostal recession and may also be using accessory muscles for respiration. Another sign of increased respiratory effort is flaring of the nostrils, which is particularly seen in young children. Listen for wheeze, stridor and a cough. It is important to characterize the cough. For example, a 'barking' cough may be suggestive of croup. Stridor can indicate laryngeal or supralaryngeal obstruction (inspiratory stridor) and biphasic stridor is caused by tracheal obstruction. Note end-expiratory grunting, which is used to increase the end-expiratory pressure.

3. Record the child's respiratory rate. This varies with the age of the child.

Age	Breaths per minute
Neonate	30–50
2–5 years	24–30
5–12 years	20–24
<12 years	12–20

4. Examine the hands for:
   a. **Clubbing:** Respiratory causes of clubbing include:
      i. Suppurative lung diseases
         A. Bronchiectasis
         B. Empyema, lung abscess
      ii. Cystic fibrosis
      iii. Interstitial lung disease
      iv. Tuberculosis
      v. Bronchial carcinoma, pleural mesothelioma
      vi. Arterio-venous fistula
   b. **Peripheral cyanosis:** See the same point in the section on cardiovascular examination.

5. Examine for the pulse. In younger children (up to toddler age), the pulse is best felt brachially. In older children and adults, the radial pulse is traditionally used. Record the heart rate. The heart rate varies with age (see the table below) and emotional state of the child. In the context of a respiratory examination, tachycardia may suggest hypoxia, fever and use of β_2 agonists such as salbutamol.

Age (years)	Beats per minute
<1	110–160
2–5	95–140
5–12	80–120
>12	60–100

Offer to measure the blood pressure. See the point in the section on cardiovascular examination for a discussion on how to do this. A low blood pressure may be a sign of sepsis or development of a tension pneumothorax.

6. Examine the neck for:

    a. **Lymphadenopathy:** See section on abdominal examination.

    b. **Tracheal deviation:** This is unpleasant for the child; therefore it is important to warn him or her about what this entails. The easiest way to do this is to place your index and ring fingers on the clavicular heads and use the middle finger to determine if the trachea is central or not. Tracheal deviation may be caused by collapse or pneumonectomy (towards the side of the pathology), tension pneumothorax or large pleural effusion (away from the side of the pathology). Mediastinal masses may also cause tracheal deviation. One may note a tracheal tug where the trachea moves on inspiration. This represents an overly expanded chest caused by airway obstruction. Hyperinflation can also be detected by measuring a decreased distance between the cricoid cartilage and the suprasternal notch. These structures should normally be three to four finger-breadths apart.

    c. **JVP:** The JVP may be examined in older children as in adults. Ask the child to turn his or her head to the left side. If the head is turned too far over the sternocleidomastoid becomes prominent and the JVP becomes difficult to see. In these cases it may be easier to see the JVP with the neck extended backwards. The JVP can be seen along the line of the internal jugular vein along the border of the sternocleidomastoid (from between the two heads of the sternocleidomastoid to the earlobe). If the JVP is low, it may not be seen, and if it is high, it may be flickering at the earlobe. The JVP is measured from the sternal angle vertically upwards and can be up to 4 cm. The JVP waveform has several characteristics. The A wave is seen in atrial contraction and may be absent in atrial fibrillation. Giant A waves, or cannon A waves, can be seen in complete heart block; V waves are caused by ventricular systole against a closed valve. If this is prominent, there is likely to be tricuspid regurgitation. The JVP may also be raised due to a tension pneumothorax or to a large pulmonary embolus. A non-pulsatile and raised JVP is indicative of superior vena cava obstruction (e.g. secondary to lymphoma or compression by an adjacent lung carcinoma). Other signs of superior vena cava obstruction may include swelling of the face and arms and distended neck and chest veins.

7. Examine the eyes for any evidence of anaemia (conjunctival pallor). In the mouth, bluish discolouration of the tongue and mucous membranes suggests central cyanosis. This is best seen by asking the child to lift the tongue to the roof of the mouth.

8. Examine for features of congenital syndromes. Scars can also provide clues, for example sternotomy or thoracotomy scars. Look for current or

healed drain or vascular access sites. Note the age of the scars and if they appear healthy. Observe the chest wall movements and whether they are symmetrical. One may note chest wall deformities such as pectus carinatum (pigeon chest) caused by a prominent sternum. Most often this is caused by poorly controlled childhood asthma or by rickets. Pectus excavatum (hollow chest) is caused by a depressed sternum. This is caused by abnormal development. In children with asthma, the anterior–posterior diameter of the chest is increased in relation to the lateral diameter (barrel chest). The child may also have spinal abnormalities such as kyphosis (increased anterior curvature) and scoliosis (increased lateral curvature) of the spine. Kyphoscoliosis involves a combination of the two deformities.

9. It is important to assess expansion of the upper chest in younger children, and of the upper and lower chest in the adolescent. Upper chest expansion is assessed by placing your hands flat on the child's upper chest and asking him or her to take a deep breath in and out. To assess expansion in the lower chest place your hands around the lower chest with your thumbs in the middle. Ask the child to take a deep breath in and out. On inspiration the thumbs should move an equal distance away from each other, 3–5 cm in school-age children. Reduced expansion can be caused by collapse, pleural effusion, consolidation or a pneumothorax. If the chest expansion is poor overall the lung disease may be more widespread such as in asthma.

10. Palpate for the apex beat. The apex beat should be felt in the fourth (<7 years old) or fifth ICS (>7 years old) in the mid-clavicular line. This may not be palpable in 40% of people, particularly obese children or those with hyperinflation. If this is displaced, possible underlying pathologies include mediastinal shift. A heave felt at the left sternal edge suggests right ventricular hypertrophy, possibly secondary to pulmonary hypertension.

11. Percussion is generally not performed on children younger than toddler age. Percuss (see Abdominal examination section for technique) the anterior chest over the lung apices (above the clavicle), over the clavicle itself (mid-clavicle as the shoulder muscles can cause dullness) and at the following three locations: upper, middle and lower chest. Each percussion should be directly compared with the opposite side. One should also percuss the axilla in the same manner (upper, middle and lower). Percussion of the posterior chest should also be performed away from the midline in order to avoid the spine and paravertebral structures. Normally percussion is resonant. Dullness to percussion suggests collapse or consolidation. Pleural effusions produce a 'stony dull' percussion note. Hyperresonant percussion indicates hyperinflation such as in asthma or a pneumothorax.

12. Using the diaphragm of the stethoscope, auscultate the chest (the bell of the stethoscope can be used above the clavicles). Auscultation can be performed in the same areas that percussion has taken place. Ask the child to

take deep breaths in and out through his or her mouth each time he or she feels the stethoscope on his or her chest. Auscultation in one area should be directly compared with the opposite side. Normal breath sounds are described as vesicular (inspiration is twice as long as expiration with no gap between the two). Reduced air entry may occur with obesity, pleural effusion, collapse, consolidation or a pneumothorax. Ask the child to cough if the breath sounds are reduced. If the cough becomes more audible, this suggests obstruction of the airways by secretions. Bronchial breathing is described as sounding similar to the breath sounds heard over the trachea. Unlike vesicular breathing, there is a pause between inspiration and expiration and both are of similar duration. This is heard over areas of consolidated lung and also at the top of a pleural effusion.

13. Ask the child to say 'ninety nine', if he or she can, each time he or she feels the stethoscope on his or her chest. This is to test for vocal resonance. Vocal resonance occurs in a consolidated lung. In a normal lung, only the low pitched components are heard. If there is effusion or collapse, the numbers are muffled. In consolidation, the numbers are clearly heard. Crackles may also be heard. In children, this is likely to be due to pneumonia, bronchiectasis or interstitial lung disease, although the latter is rare. Wheeze is typically heard during expiration. Inspiratory wheeze suggests severe airway narrowing. A wheeze has a musical quality to it and may suggest obstruction or asthma. It is customary to complete examination of the anterior chest prior to moving onto the posterior chest. The sequence of palpation, percussion and auscultation can then be repeated on the posterior chest as described above in each section.

14. Offer to perform a peak flow meter test. If this is agreed to, remember to take the best of three readings.

15. Thank the parents and, if appropriate, the child. Provide a summary of your examination findings and suggest further investigations. For example:

> I examined Amelie who is 5 years old and has presented with a chronic cough productive of sputum. On inspection, I noted that there was a sputum pot containing green sputum at the bedside. The patient looked tachypnoeic at rest with a respiratory rate of 34 breaths per minute. On general inspection, I noted that Amelie's fingers were clubbed. There were no other peripheral stigmata of respiratory disease. Chest expansion was equal bilaterally. On percussion, I noted dullness to percussion, and both inspiratory crackles and expiratory wheeze, bibasally. Vocal resonance was also reduced bilaterally.
>
> These findings would be consistent with a diagnosis of suppurative lung disease, possibly cystic fibrosis.
>
> To complete my examination, I would like to send the sputum for microscopy and culture, perform a peak flow, record the oxygen saturations and temperature and order a CXR.

1. What further investigations may be appropriate to perform following a respiratory examination?

To complete a respiratory examination, the acronym **SPOT-X** is used to list the most important investigations: **S**putum, **P**eak flow, **O**xygen, **T**emperature and **C**XR. Further investigations to complete the examination will depend on the underlying diagnosis obtained from a thorough history and examination, and can be stratified as follows:

a. Immediate bedside tests
   i. Sputum (in older children)
   ii. Nasopharyngeal aspirates
   iii. O_2 saturations
   iv. Peak flow assessment
   v. Arterial blood gas
      A. Painful, so consider carefully in children who are not sedated and ventilated
   vi. Lung function tests
b. Laboratory tests
   i. Blood tests
c. Imaging
   i. Chest X-ray
   ii. CT (high-resolution CT)
   iii. PET
   iv. Staging scans
d. Invasive tests
   i. Broncho-alveolar lavage
   ii. Biopsy
   iii. Bronchoscopy

Peripheral neurological examination

'Barney is 4 years old. He has had delay in reaching his motor milestones. Please perform a peripheral neurological examination of both the upper and lower limbs.'

(Note that in reality in an OSCE, you will most likely be asked to examine *either* the upper or lower limbs.)

Score Sheet

Scores: 1 = Not attempted; 2 = Attempted, unsatisfactory; 3 = Attempted, satisfactory

Action	1	2	3
1. Performs introduction, washes hands			
2. Performs a general observation of the child, mentions doing a brief developmental assessment			

Continued

Action	1	2	3
3. Examines gait			
4. Examines tone			
5. Assesses for pronator drift			
6. Assesses power			
7. Examines the reflexes			
8. Examines coordination			
9. Examines sensation			
10. Summarized findings and suggests further investigations			
Overall score		/30	

1. Remember **WIIPPE: W**ash hands, **I**ntroduction, **I**dentity, **P**ermission, **P**osition, **E**xposure.
2. In a neurological examination, it is important to perform a quick assessment of the developmental milestones the child has reached and to compare him or her to the expected development rate (see Developmental examination section). A great deal of information for both the developmental and the neurological examination can come from watching a child. This may be through the child's social interaction or by watching the child at play. The latter observation provides a crude assessment of gross motor function as well as other modalities; as a child reaches for his or her toys this suggests that he or she does not have underlying cerebellar or proprioceptive pathology. Similar observations can be made during the examination. For example, if a child tries to fight off the examiner, this suggests that he or she has good power. If the expected developmental milestones have not been reached, one should attempt to elucidate the underlying cause.

   In infants, the important things to note are whether the child is irritable, floppy or stiff, and whether his or her movements are symmetrical. There are multiple causes for a floppy child. The main pathologies are listed in the box below.

   Observe for areas of increased muscle bulk. In Duchenne muscular dystrophy, one may note pseudohypertrophy of the calf. Conversely,

> **CAUSES OF A 'FLOPPY CHILD'**
> Cerebral palsy
> Spinal cord injury
> Myaesthenia gravis
> Myopathies
> Dystrophies
> Ehlers Danlos syndrome
> Benign infant hypotonia

there may be evidence of wasting. As a general rule, distal muscle wasting suggests a neuropathy and proximal muscle wasting suggests a myopathy. One may note fasciculations. These can be best seen on the tongue but may be seen elsewhere.

3. If the child is able to walk, observe him or her walking back and forth across the room. When children begin to walk they usually have a broad-based gait. However, this may also suggest cerebellar ataxia where the child has a broad unsteady gait and usually falls towards the side of the underlying lesion. The usual gait is in a heel-toe pattern. If a child walks in a toe-heel pattern this may be normal. However, it can also suggest corticospinal pathology, neuropathy, spinal pathology or the tight Achilles tendon in muscular dystrophy. If it is difficult to establish the mode of walking, ask to look at the child's shoes for the pattern of wear. With a hemiplegic gait, the child drags the leg around as he or she walks, scraping the foot on the ground (circumduction). This is more obvious when the child attempts to run. If a child has proximal muscle weakness, for example with muscular dystrophy, he or she may display a 'waddling gait'.

If there are signs of weakness, ask the child to lie down and then stand up. If the child is below 3 years, he or she will turn onto his or her front in order to do this. If this persists in an older child, this is a sign of muscular weakness, such as in muscular dystrophy, or hypotonia. This is similar to Gower's sign – seen in Duchenne's – where the child uses his or her hands to climb up his or her legs in order to stand up.

4. Tone can be assessed in a number of ways. Testing for head lag involves lifting the child from a lying position by his or her wrists. The child should be momentarily able to hold his or her head. Head lag is normal up to 4 months of age. Testing for vertical suspension involves holding the child under each armpit. The child should be able to support himself/ herself in this position, but if he or she is hypotonic, the child will slip through. Testing for ventral suspension involves holding the child in the prone position on the palm of your hand. The child should extend his or her back and hips while flexing the arms and legs and lifting the head. While the child is lying down, he or she normally displays adduction at his or her hips, but in a hypotonic child there is complete abduction of the hips. This is likened to the position of a 'pithed frog'. In a hypotonic child, it is important to ascertain whether or not there is weakness (see the point below on power). Hypotonia with weakness would imply a peripheral cause, whereas a lack of weakness suggests a chromosomal abnormality or a central pathology.

Tone in the older child can be assessed as for an adult. Ask the child to relax his or her arm and passively move the joints of the upper limb. Then move onto assessing for tone in the leg. This is best assessed by rolling the leg on the bed and then putting a hand behind the knee and lifting it rapidly. If the heel easily leaves the bed when the knee is pulled up, this is a sign of spasticity and the opposite is true for flaccidity. If the child is finding it difficult to relax, aim to distract the child with a toy or by questioning him or her, for example, about a typical school day. Clonus is best assessed at the ankle. Dorsiflex the ankle briskly and feel for downbeats of the foot. A total of more than three clonus beats is abnormal. Pyramidal pathology manifests as increased tone in pronation of the forearms, the adductors and internal rotators of the hip, together with clonus. This may occur in cerebral palsy. Another cause of increased tone which is important not to miss is myotonia. This occurs when the muscles fail to relax after an active movement. For example, the child cannot let go after shaking hands.

5. Assess for pronator drift. Ask the child to hold the arms out in front of him or her with the palms facing upwards, and to close his or her eyes. Central lesions will cause pronation with a downward drift. In a cerebellar lesion, there is pronation with an upwards drift. If the child has a peripheral neuropathy, he or she may display pseudoathetosis where the fingers will display 'searching movements'.

6. Power is difficult to assess in babies. The best way to assess for this is to observe the movements against gravity. After 4 years, power can be formally assessed.

   a. **Upper limb:** Ask the child to put his or her arms up, elbows at the side, like a chicken, and to stop you pushing the arms down. Ask the child to put his or her arms up in front like a boxer and first push you away and then pull you towards him or her. Next ask the child to put his or her arms out straight and cock the wrist back, then stop you pushing the wrist down and pushing the wrist up. Ask the child to keep the arms outstretched and ask him or her to stop you pushing his or her fingers down and pushing his or her fingers up. Finally, ask the child to spread his or her fingers and, using your index finger and little finger, ask the child to stop you pushing the index and little finger in and out. In each case, test power at each joint separately and use your other hand to provide stability just above the joint that is being tested. For example, when testing the fingers, stabilize the wrist joint to ensure the power being tested is only that of the fingers. The muscles and nerves corresponding to each action are listed in the table below.

Action	Muscle	Nerve root	Nerve
Shoulder abduction	Deltoid	C5	Axillary
Elbow flexion	Biceps	C5, 6	Musculocutaneous
Elbow extension	Triceps	C7	Radial
Wrist flexion	Flexor carpi radialis, flexor carpi ulnaris	C8	Median, ulnar
Wrist extension	Extensor carpi radialis, extensor carpi ulnaris	C7	Radial

Continued

Action	Muscle	Nerve root	Nerve
Finger flexion	Flexor digitorum superficialis and profundus	C8	Median, ulnar
Finger extension	Extensor digitorum	C7	Radial (posterior interosseus)
Finger abduction	Dorsal interosseus	T1	Ulnar
Finger adduction	Palmar interosseus	T1	Ulnar
Thumb abduction	Abductor pollicis brevis	T1	Median

Power should be recorded according to the MRC power scale in the box below.

MRC SCALE

5 = normal power
4 = submaximal power
3 = movement against gravity but not against resistance
2 = movement when gravity is eliminated
1 = flicker
0 = no movement

b. **Lower limb:** In the lower limb, ask the child to straighten his or her leg and lift it up from the bed and then try to stop you from pushing it down/pulling it up. Ask the child to bend the knees up and then try to pull the heel into his or her bottom while you try to pull in the opposite direction; then ask him or her to try and straighten his or her leg out against your resistance. Next ask him or her to straighten his or her legs and stop you pushing his or her foot down and then stop you from pushing his or her foot upwards. Finally, ask him or her to stop you pushing his or her big toe down and then from pulling it up. In each case, test power at each joint separately and use your other hand to provide stability just above the joint that is being tested. The muscles and nerves corresponding to each action are listed in the table below.

Action	Muscle	Nerve root	Nerve
Hip flexion	Iliopsoas	L2, 3	Lumbar sacral plexus
Hip extension	Gluteus maximus	L5, S1	Inferior gluteal nerve
Knee extension	Quadriceps femoris	L3, 4	Femoral nerve
Knee flexion	Hamstrings	L5, S1	Sciatic nerve
Dorsiflexion	Anterior tibialis	L4, 5	Deep peroneal nerve
Plantarflexion	Gastrocnemius	S1	Posterior tibial nerve
Big toe extension	Extensor hallucis longus	L5	Deep peroneal nerve

7. Test for reflexes in the neonate with your fingertip. In older children a tendon hammer may be used. It is essential to relax the child. Brisk reflexes may occur when the child is anxious. They may also suggest an upper motor neuron (UMN) lesion. Absent reflexes may be due to poor examiner technique or to lower motor neuron (LMN) lesions. The following reflexes should be tested: biceps, triceps, supinator, knee and ankle jerks, and the plantar reflex.

a. **Upper limb:** To elicit the biceps reflex, ask the child to place his or her arm across his or her abdomen. Place your index finger on the biceps tendon and strike your finger with a tendon hammer. For the triceps reflex, draw the arm across the chest holding the wrist with the elbow at 90° and strike the triceps tendon directly. For the supinator reflex, place the child's hand on his or her abdomen. Place your index finger on the radial tuberosity and strike your finger. Reflexes are graded from very brisk to absent as illustrated in the box below.

> **Grading reflexes**
> 0 = absent
> ± = present only with reinforcement
> 1+ = present but depressed
> 2+ = normal
> 3+ = increased
> 4+ = clonus

b. **Lower limb:** For the knee jerk reflex, place your arm under the knee and strike the patella tendon with the tendon hammer. For the ankle jerk reflex, turn the foot out to the side with the ankle at 90° and strike the Achilles tendon directly. The muscles and nerve corresponding to each reflex are listed in the tables below. If the child is having difficultly relaxing, it is possible to use reinforcement techniques, if the child is able. When the upper limb reflexes are being tested, the child is asked to clench his or her teeth on the count of three. Similarly, when the lower limb reflexes are being tested, the child is asked to clasp his or her hands together and attempt to pull them apart, again on the count of three.

Reflex	Muscle	Nerve root	Nerve
Biceps	Biceps	C5, 6	Musculocutaneous
Triceps	Triceps	C7	Radial
Supinator	Brachioradialis	C6	Radial
Finger jerk, Hoffman's sign	Flexor digitorum profundus and superficialis	C8	Median and ulnar
Knee jerk	Quadriceps	L3, L4	Femoral nerve
Ankle jerk	Gastrocnemius	L5, S1	Tibial nerve

UMN lesion
- Increased tone, brisk reflexes, up-going plantar reflex

LMN lesion
- Hypotonia, decreased or absent reflexes, wasting, fasciculations

The final reflex to test for is the plantar reflex. In children under the age of one, this is unpleasant and equivocal. In order to test for the plantar reflex, gently draw a pointed stick up the lateral border of the foot and across the ball of the foot. Keep a close eye on the big toe. Flexion of the big toe is a normal response. If the big toe extends while all the other toes flex, this is a positive plantar reflex. A positive response suggests UMN pathology. N.B. If the big toe and the other toes extend and the ankle dorsiflexes, this is more likely to be due to withdrawal.

At this point in the examination one should be able to assess whether the pathology is indicative of UMN or LMN pathology. The box above highlights the distinguishing features.

8. Coordination can be assessed in a number of ways. This can be assessed through play. If building blocks are available, the child can be asked to build one block on top of another. Alternatively, he or she can be asked to do up and undo buttons, to draw, write or copy images. After the age of two, the child can be asked to touch his or her nose and then touch your finger. This can be performed using a teddy bear, asking the child to touch the bear's nose, to engage the child. The finger-to-nose test elicits cerebellar dysfunction, specifically looking for an intention tremor and past pointing. Another test of coordination involves asking the child to touch each finger to his or her thumb in turn. The lower limbs can similarly be assessed opportunistically, for example, by asking the child to hop, stand on one leg and walk heel-to-toe. These tasks test for coordination as well as proprioceptive abilities.

9. When testing for sensation, the ability to withdraw to tickling is a good screening test. If a sensory deficit is suspected, more formal testing should be performed in an older child, as in adults. Ask the child to close his or her eyes and to say 'yes' when he or she can feel light touch (using a piece of cotton wool). Sensation should be tested dermatomally in the upper and lower limb.

10. Investigations to complete the examination will depend on the underlying diagnosis obtained from a thorough history and examination. A general answer may include completing a cranial nerve examination and formally testing the other modalities of sensation, such as pin prick and temperature, as well as proprioception and vibration. Summarize your findings. For example:

I examined Barney, who is 4 years old and has presented with difficulty walking. On inspection of his walking, I noted that he had a waddling gait. His calves appeared hypertrophied. He demonstrated a positive Gower's sign. On examination, tone was normal. Power was reduced at the pelvic girdle (4/5) but the remainder of the upper and lower limb was normal. Coordination was normal in the upper limbs, but I was unable to test coordination in the lower limbs as this would have been confounded by the weakness. I was able to elicit reflexes throughout. Sensation was grossly intact.

These findings would be consistent with a diagnosis of muscular dystrophy, most likely Duchenne muscular dystrophy.

To complete my examination, I would like to perform a cranial nerve examination and formally test the other modalities of sensation such as pin prick and temperature, as well as proprioception and vibration.

Cranial nerve examination

'Holly is 7 years old. She has had a recent viral infection and her parents have noticed facial asymmetry. Please perform a cranial nerve examination.'

Score Sheet

Scores: 1 = Not attempted; 2 = Attempted, unsatisfactory; 3 = Attempted, satisfactory

Action	1	2	3
1. Performs introduction, washes hands			
2. Offers to test olfactory nerve (or asks question regarding sense of smell)			
3. Assesses visual acuity, visual fields and pupillary reflexes			
4. Assesses eye movement			
5. Tests the trigeminal nerve (motor and sensory components)			
6. Assesses facial movement			
7. Assesses hearing			
8. Performs a test for the glossopharyngeal and vagus nerves			
9. Assesses accessory nerve function			
10. Assesses hypoglossal nerve function			
11. Summarizes findings and suggests further investigations			
Overall score	/33		

1. Use **WIIPPE: W**ash hands, **I**ntroduction, **I**dentity, **P**ermission, **P**osition, **E**xposure. Ideally the child should be seated in a chair. Below the age of 4 years old, it may not be possible to assess all aspects of a cranial nerve examination. A great deal of information can be gained from observing the child. It may be difficult to perform the cranial nerve examination in order and as such one often needs to be opportunistic. The manner in which to examine each of the cranial nerves in neonates and infants versus a child over the age of 4 years is described below.

2. **Olfactory nerve I:** Olfactory dysfunction is rare in paediatrics but can be tested for in older children by asking whether there has been any change in their sense of smell and taste and also by formally using smelling salts (peppermint, camphor, rosewater and ammonia).

3. **Optic nerve II:** The components of acuity can be remembered by the acronym AFRO (acuity, fields, reflexes and opthalmoscopy).

    a. **Acuity:** It is difficult to assess acuity in a neonate but one can check gross vision by observing the ability to fix on objects or faces. In an older child, visual acuity can be assessed formally using a Snellen chart. If a Snellen chart is not available, a newspaper can be used. Ask the child to cover one eye and then read a line of text. Cover the other eye and repeat. Ensure that the text the child is asked to read is the same size in each case. If the child is unable to read, ask them to count your fingers. If they are unable to do this, assess whether the child can see hand movements or perceive light.

    b. **Visual fields:** In an older child, one can also assess for visual fields. Sit so that you are at the same level as the child. Ask the child to cover one eye and you do the same with the opposite eye. Bring a moving finger in at an oblique angle from the top right/left and bottom right/left and ask the child when he or she can first see the finger moving. Ensure that you test all four quadrants. Formal visual field testing is performed with Goldman perimetry.

    c. **Reflexes:** *Pupillary reflex:* the afferent pathway is from the optic nerve and the efferent pathway is from the oculomotor nerve. This is tested for by shining a light into the eye and observing for pupillary constriction in both the ipsilateral eye (direct reflex) and the contralateral eye (consensual reflex). Note asymmetry of the pupils at this point. If this is the case, then a cover test can be performed (this will not be discussed here). *Accommodation reflex:* the afferent pathway arises in the frontal lobe and the efferent pathway is from the oculomotor nerve. Place your finger 10 cm from the child's nose and ask him or her to look into the corner of the room and then at your finger. The pupils should constrict.

    d. **Ophthalmoscopy:** This is difficult in a young child but one can test for the red reflex which, is absent, may suggest a cataract or retinoblastoma.

4. **Oculomotor nerve III, trochlear nerve IV and abducens nerve VI:** One has to use creativity in assessing eye movements in a younger child. Use a toy and move it through horizontal and vertical planes while observing eye movements. In an older child, hold the chin steady and ask them to follow your finger with their eyes. Move in an H shape, observe for nystagmus and ask the child if they can see double at any point. Nystagmus suggests cerebellar disease. Be aware of nystagmus at the extremes of lateral gaze, which is normal.

5. **Trigeminal nerve V:** In infants and neonates, test for the rooting response. Touch lightly at the corner of the mouth. This should cause the

mouth to open and the head to rotate in the direction of the stimulus. Test for the motor component of the trigeminal nerve in an older child by asking them to clench their teeth while you feel for the contraction of the masseter and temporalis muscles. Ask the child to waggle the jaw from side to side against resistance. Next test for the sensory component of the trigeminal nerve. Ask the child to close their eyes and then ask them to say 'yes' each time they feel light touch (forehead, cheek and chin on both sides). It is also important to assess for trigeminal reflexes (or in an OSCE, just offer to do so). *Jaw jerk*: the afferent and efferent pathways are made up by the trigeminal nerves. Ask the child to hang their mouth open loosely. Place a finger on their chin and then strike your finger with a tendon hammer. *Corneal reflex* (this is not usually performed): the afferent pathway is from the trigeminal nerve and the efferent pathway is from the facial nerve. To test for a corneal reflex, touch the cornea with a piece of cotton wool to elicit a blink.

6. **Facial nerve VII:** In infants and neonates, observe the symmetry of facial movements. Look for asymmetry especially when the child smiles or cries. In an older child, test the muscles of facial expression by asking them to raise the eyebrows, close the eyes tightly, puff their cheeks out and show you their teeth. Taste, although not routinely done, can be tested by dipping a cotton wool bud in a sugar or saline solution and then applying this to each side of the tongue (anterior two-thirds).

7. **Vestibulocochlear nerve VIII:** Ask the parents if there have been any issues with hearing (although this screening question may miss unilateral hearing loss). In a neonate or infant, use a tuning fork to grossly assess hearing. Strike a tuning fork and place it next to the child's ear. The child should turn towards the sound. In an older child, hearing can be grossly assessed by rubbing your fingers next to one ear to mask that ear while whispering a number into the other ear. If the child is unable to repeat the numbers, then Rinne's and Weber's test may be performed (see boxes below). These differentiate between conductive deafness (failure of

---

RINNE'S TEST

Hold a 516-Hz tuning fork against the mastoid process (bone conduction) and then 2.5 cm from the external auditory meatus (air conduction). Ask which is louder.

Normally the transmission through the outer and middle ear is better than through bone to the cochlea which bypasses the middle ear, and so in normal ears air conduction is better than bone conduction.

In conductive deafness, because of problems in the outer and middle ear, bone conduction is better.

In sensorineural deafness, there is impairment whether through air or bone, so Rinne's test does not help elicit this.

WEBER'S TEST

Hold a 516-Hz tuning fork in the middle of the forehead. The sound is usually heard equally in both ears.

In conductive deafness, the sound localizes to the affected ear (due to lack of competitive sounds that would normally be heard on that side).

In sensorineural deafness, the sound lateralizes to the normal ear.

transmission of sound from the outer or middle ear to the cochlea) and sensorineural deafness (diseases of the cochlea, cochlear nuclei and their supranuclear connections). Both of these tests need to be performed to reach a firm conclusion.

The note sounded by a 512-Hz tuning fork is an octave above middle C.

8. **Glossopharyngeal nerve IX, vagus nerve X:** These nerves are usually assessed together. If the infant or neonate is crying or has their mouth open, look at the position of the uvula and palate. If the palate is drooping on one side and the uvula is deviated, this suggests vagus nerve pathology. Insert a finger into child's mouth. The child should respond by sucking your finger. If the parents say that there has been any difficulty with feeding this would suggest there may be underlying neurological problems. In an older child, ask them to say 'aah' and again observe the palate and uvula. Hoarseness of the voice may suggest a laryngeal nerve lesion. Although the reflexes are not usually performed one may be asked how to carry out a gag reflex. *Gag reflex*: the afferent pathway is from the glossopharyngeal nerve and efferent pathway is from the vagus nerve. Touch the pharyngeal wall behind the pillars of the fauces. Watch the uvula; it should lift following the stimulus.

9. **Accessory nerve XI:** In infants and neonates, weakness of the trapezius and sternocleidomastoid will be detected through inability to turn the head when testing for the rooting response (see above). In an older child, ask the child to shrug his or her shoulders up against resistance (trapezius) and to turn his or her head to the left or the right against resistance (sternocleidomastoid).

10. **Hypoglossal nerve XII:** Observe for atrophy or fasciculations of the tongue. Ask the child to stick his or her tongue out, looking for deviation. If the tongue does deviate, it is towards the side of the lesion.

11. Thank the parents and, if appropriate, the child. Provide a summary of your examination findings and suggest further investigations. For example:

> *I examined Holly who is 7 years old and presented with facial asymmetry. On examination there was an obvious left-sided facial droop. Cranial nerve testing was normal apart from examination of the facial nerve. There was obvious weakness of orbicularis oris (muscle around the mouth) and orbicularis ocularis (muscle that closes the*

eyelids) but sparing of frontalis (forehead muscle) suggesting that this is a lower motor neurone lesion.

Given the recent viral illness, these findings would be consistent with a diagnosis of post-infective Bell's palsy.

To complete my examination, I would like to perform an ear examination, peripheral nerve examination and formally test the other modalities of sensation such as pin prick and temperature, as well as proprioception and vibration.

Ear and throat examination

'Finley is 3 years old. He has been feeling unwell for the last 2 days with a fever, and now has pain in his left ear. Please perform an examination of his ears and throat.'

Score Sheet

Scores: 1 = Not attempted; 2 = Attempted, unsatisfactory; 3 = Attempted, satisfactory

Action	1	2	3
1. Performs introduction, washes hands			
2. Chooses the correct speculum size for the otoscope			
3. Positions the child appropriately for ear examination			
4. Examines the external ears			
5. Examines the ears with the otoscope			
6. Positions the child appropriately for throat examination			
7. Examines the teeth and throat			
8. Examines the cervical lymph nodes			
9. Summarizes findings			
Overall score		/27	

Ear examination

1. Use the acronym **WIIPPE**: **W**ash hands, **I**ntroduction, **I**dentity, **P**ermission, **P**osition, **E**xposure.
2. In order to look inside the ears ensure that the otoscope has a speculum which is large enough for a snug fit within the ear canal. In a newborn, this is usually 2 mm; in younger children use 4 mm; and in older children, use 5 mm. In order to put the child at ease, carry out a mock examination on a teddy bear and use distraction techniques, for example, with toys.
3. Position the child on the mother's knee facing sideways. Ask the parent to put an arm across the child's arm and body.
4. Inspect the external ear looking for discharge and erythema. Look behind the ear for a swelling, which may indicate mastoiditis.
5. Hold the otoscope head between your thumb and index and middle fingers using the back of your hand to act as a support against

the child's face. This is to ensure that the otoscope is stable should the child move. Gently pull the pinna upwards and backwards. Aim the speculum of the otoscope towards the front and top of the opposite pinna. Once the eardrum is visualized, look for the landmarks such as the handle of the malleus as well as erythema, discharge and swelling. In order to minimize distress, always start with the normal ear.

Throat examination

6. The best way to do this examination in a child who is likely to be uncooperative is to place them on the mother's knee. Ask the mother to put one hand across the child's head and one hand across their arms.

7. Use a spatula in young children and try to examine the tonsils, pharynx, palate and tonsils as quickly as possible. Look particularly for redness, pus, swelling and petechiae. Look at the teeth for caries and any abnormalities of the gums. In older children, a spatula may not be required.

8. To complete the examination of the throat, palpate the lymph nodes in the neck as previously described.

9. Thank the parents and, if appropriate, the child. Provide a summary of your examination findings. For example:

> *I examined Finley who is 3 years old and presented with a recent history of feeling unwell with a fever and left ear pain. On examination, the external left ear was normal. There was evidence of inflammation of the left tympanic membrane, but no evidence of perforation or discharge. The right ear was normal. Examination of the throat was also unremarkable, and there was no palpably cervical lymphadenopathy.*
>
> *These findings would be consistent with a diagnosis of acute otitis media.*

DATA INTERPRETATION

Growth charts

'Katie is a 23-month-old baby born at 36 weeks, who has presented to clinic as her head circumference remains below the second centile. Her height and weight are in the tenth centile.'

The UK and World Health Organization growth charts cover boys and girls from ages 0 to 4 years, and are available on the Royal College of Paediatrics and Child Health website. You should familiarize yourself with them and be comfortable using these to read off centiles given specific measurements.

Questions

1. Describe the normal sequence of events in head growth.
   Head growth occurs in the first 24 months of life. By the age of five, a child's head size will be 80% of that of an adult. The anterior and posterior fontanelles close at 12–18 months and 8 weeks, respectively.

2. What is the definition of microcephaly?
   This is a head circumference below the second centile.

3. What are the common causes of microcephaly?
   Microcephaly may be familial, or can be caused by congenital infection, or as a sequel to hypoxic ischaemic encephalopathy.

4. What is the definition of macrocephaly?
   This is a head circumference above the 98th centile.

5. What are the common causes of macrocephaly?
   Macrocephaly may be familial or caused by raised intracranial pressure, hydrocephalus, aubdural haematoma or storage disorders.

'Anran is a 4-year-old child who is small for his age. His parents are concerned as he does not seem to be growing at the same rate as the other children in his class, and he is being bullied.'

Questions

1. How is height measured in children?
   Up to 2 years, the length of the child lying down is measured. At 2 years and above the standing height of the child is measured.

2. What is the definition of short stature?
   Short stature is defined as a height below the 0.4th centile.

3. What are the causes of short stature?
   a. Familial
   b. Constitutional delay of growth and puberty
      Delayed puberty may run in the family but the child will usually reach their target height.
   c. Prematurity/intrauterine growth restriction
      One-third of those children who are born prematurely or who suffer intrauterine growth restriction will remain short.
   d. Chromosomal disorder
      Most chromosomal disorders such as Down's syndrome are diagnosed at birth, but syndromes such as Turner's syndrome may be difficult to diagnose.
   e. Endocrine
      Growth hormone deficiency, hypothyroidism and corticosteroid excess.
   f. Nutritional
      This may be due to dietary deficiency. Other conditions that can cause nutritional deficiency include coeliac disease, Crohn's disease and cystic fibrosis.
   g. Psychosocial
      Physical and emotional abuse can lead to children whose growth is impaired. When placed in a nurturing environment, the child will usually display a catch-up of growth.

4. How is the target height calculated in children where it is thought that short stature is familial?

The mid-parental height is first calculated. In boys, this is:

[(mother's height (cm) + father's height (cm))/2] + 6.5 (cm)

In girls, this is:

[(mother's height (cm) + father's height (cm))/2] − 6.5 (cm).

The target range is the mid-parental height ±10 cm.

5. What are the causes of tall stature?
   a. Familial
   b. Obesity
      Overeating in childhood may fuel growth.
   c. Endocrine
      Growth hormone excess, hyperthyroidism, excess sex steroids
   d. Chromosomal disorder
      Marfan's syndrome and Klinefelter's syndrome
   e. Tall stature at birth
      Maternal diabetes

Recognition of abuse

Take some time to familiarize yourself with images available online that are relevant to this subject. Common images you may be expected to identify include:

a. Marks on the hands, legs or face from striking
b. Scalds with patterns suspicious of non-accidental injury
c. Mongolian blue spots (a normal feature)
d. Torn frenulum of the upper lip

Questions

1. What are the different types of child abuse?

   Child abuse may be physical, emotional, sexual, be caused by neglect or by Munchausen's syndrome by proxy (symptoms are fabricated by the carer). A child can present with evidence of more than one form of abuse.

2. What features in a history would make you suspicious that a child was being abused?

   The carer may provide a history that is unlikely to have resulted in the observed injury. There may have been a delay in reporting the incident. Each time the history is taken, there may be inconsistencies apparent from the carer themselves or others involved in the care of the child. The injuries may be inconsistent with the age of the child. The carers may not respond appropriately; for example, they may seem unconcerned or become unnecessarily aggressive. The child may continue to re-present with recurrent injuries.

3. What would make you suspicious about bruising in a child?

Suspect non-accidental injury if there is bruising that is not caused by a medical condition (e.g. coagulation disorder) and which cannot be explained by the history offered. For example:

a. Bruising in a child who is not independently mobile

b. Multiple areas of bruising that are of a similar size and shape ('pattern bruising')

c. Bruising in non-bony areas (cheeks, ears, buttocks)

d. Fingertip bruising, bruising on the neck that looks like strangulation marks

4. How might you detect a non-accidental head injury?

There may be no external signs of head injury in a shaken baby but there may be clues. The child may present with irritability, seizures or reduced oral intake. On examination, he or she may have an increased head circumference with or without a bulging fontanelle. On fundoscopy, there may be evidence of retinal haemorrhages. Apnoea, seizures and 'floppiness' could all be a presenting feature.

5. What would make you suspicious about burns/scalds in a child?

Accidental scalds are usually asymmetrical with splash marks. Deliberate scalds are symmetrical and may scald the back which would be uncommon in an accidental injury. Some burns may be typical of their aetiology, such as cigarette burns.

6. What would make you suspicious about fractures in a child?

Posterior rib fractures in children under 30 months are usually caused by squeezing. Have a high index of suspicion for metaphyseal fractures and spiral fractures. Multiple fractures of different ages could be indicative of abuse.

7. How might neglect, emotional abuse, Münchausen by proxy and sexual abuse present?

Neglect may present with poor hygiene, lack of emotional attachment with the carer, delay in development as well as poor attendance at school and for immunizations. Emotional abuse usually results in behavioural disturbances. In fabricated illnesses, the carer may put blood in the vomit, stool in the urine or sugar in the urine. Sexual abuse must be suspected if a child presents with genital trauma or infection, overly sexual behaviour or unexplained pregnancy.

8. What medical conditions should you be aware of that could mimic child abuse?

Bruising may be caused by clotting disorders such as immune thrombocytopaenic purpura. Multiple fractures of different ages can be secondary to osteogenesis imperfecta. In this case, children may also have blue sclera. Copper deficiency may also cause fractures. Scalded skin syndrome, or bullous impetigo, may cause lesions that look like burns or scalds. Mongolion blue spots have been mistaken for bruising due to non-accidental injury.

9. How would you escalate your suspicion of physical child abuse?
   If you have a suspicion of child abuse, you must inform the paediatric consultant on call and contact social services. Check if the child is already on the child protection register. Ensure documentation is clear and accurate as well as dated, timed and signed as medical notes are used as evidence. Take photos of any visible injuries. The child should be placed in a place of safety for protection and further assessment. Siblings also must be examined for evidence of abuse, and their safety should be taken into consideration.

10. What investigations should be performed in a child who is suspected as being a victim of physical abuse?
    A skeletal survey should be performed in children under 2 years of age in order to identify current as well as old bony injuries. A CT/MRI brain should also be performed if head injury is suspected as well as fundoscopy to look for evidence of retinal haemorrhages. An extended clotting screen and platelet count should be carried out if a child presents with extensive bruising. The extended clotting screen includes tests for factors 8, 9, 11 and 13, platelet glycoproteins, alpha-2 antiplasmin and von Willebrand factor and activity.

Spot diagnoses

Images for 'spot diagnoses' may be given to you in an OSCE. Search online to familiarize yourself with the variety of presentations. Conditions that lend themselves to spot diagnoses include:

- Down's syndrome
- Turner's syndrome
- Williams syndrome

Questions

1. List some features and late complications of Down's syndrome
   a. Facial features
      i. Flat occiput
      ii. Flat nasal bridge
      iii. Small mouth
      iv. Small ears
      v. Upslanting palpebral fissures
      vi. Epicanthic folds (fold of skin on inner edge of palpebral fissure)
   b. Other features
      i. Single palmar crease
      ii. Sandal gap toe
      iii. Clinodactyly (curved fifth finger)
      iv. Congenital heart disease

   c. Late complications
      i. Developmental delay
     ii. Cataracts
    iii. Small stature
    iv. Learning difficulties
     v. Hypothyroidism
    vi. Increased susceptibility to leukaemia
   vii. Alzheimer's disease

2. List some features of Turner's syndrome
   Alzheimer's disease
   Short stature
   Wide carrying angle
   Widely spaced nipples
   Delayed puberty
   Infertility
   Congenital heart disease (coarctation of the aorta)
   Hypothyroidism

3. List some features of Williams syndrome
   Full cheeks
   Wide mouth with full lips
   Small widely spaced teeth
   Aortic stenosis
   Learning difficulties
   Over friendliness

Rashes

In an OSCE, rashes can be presented to you as either an image or a description as part of a clinical scenario. Familiarize yourself with images of common skin conditions, including infections (e.g. chicken pox, measles, impetigo, molluscum contagiosum, hand foot and mouth disease), vascular malformations (e.g. port wine stain, strawberry naevus) and those which may be part of congenital conditions (e.g. café-au-lait spots of neurofibromatosis, cutaneous features of tuberose sclerosis).

Based on the following descriptions of rashes, decide a possible underlying diagnosis and answer the following questions.

An 8-month-old baby presents with fever, irritability, lethargy, vomiting and poor feeding. His mother has noticed a non-blanching rash on his arms and legs and soon after admission to hospital he had a witnessed seizure.

Questions

1. What is the likely diagnosis?
   The diagnosis is meningitis with sepsis until proven otherwise.

2. What are the common causative organisms of meningitis in children?

The causative organisms depend on the age of the child. In neonates, common organisms include Group B *Streptococcus*, *Listeria monocytogenes* and *Escherichia coli*. In children from 1 month to 6 years, common organisms include *Neisseria meningitides* (meningococcus), *Streptococcus pneumonia* and *Haemophilus influenzae*. In children older than 6 years, common organisms include *N. meningitides* and *S. pneumoniae*. Note that the presence of the non-blanching rash (purpura) is indicative of meningococcal (*N. meningitides*) septicaemia.

3. What investigations should be carried out?

Investigations include blood tests including FBC, clotting, U&Es (including calcium and magnesium), LFTs, CRP, glucose, blood culture and blood gas. Urine should be sent for microscopy and culture, and throat swabs should be taken. A lumbar puncture should also be performed.

4. What are the common cerebrospinal fluid (CSF) findings for bacterial, tuberculous and viral meningitis?

A CSF sample obtained from a child with bacterial meningitis is turbid in appearance. A cell count shows an increase in mainly neutrophils, with high protein levels and low glucose levels. In TB meningitis, the CSF is also turbid in appearance. Cell count shows an increase in lymphocytes, with high protein and very low glucose levels. In viral meningitis, the CSF is clear in appearance and shows an increase in lymphocytes. Protein levels may be normal or slightly raised and glucose is usually normal.

5. What is the management of bacterial meningitis in children?

Management is with immediate administration of intravenous antibiotics, usually a third-generation cephalosporin. In children below the age of 3 months, amoxycillin should be added to cover *Listeria monocytogenes*.

A 3-year-old boy presents with 6 days of fever. His eyes are red and there is evidence of skin peeling on the palms of the hands and the soles of the feet.

Questions

1. What is the likely diagnosis?

The likely diagnosis is Kawasaki's disease.

2. What are the criteria for diagnosis?

The diagnosis is made clinically. This requires a fever of more than 5 days and four out of the following five criteria: bilateral conjunctival injection, signs in the mouth (dryness, strawberry tongue), cervical lymphadenopathy, polymorphous exanthema (widespread rash) and signs in the hands/feet (desquamation, erythema, oedema).

3. What are the complications?

Complications include coronary artery aneurysms and sudden death.

4. What is the management?
Management is with IV immunoglobulins (IgA) and aspirin.

A 7-year-old boy presents with abdominal pain and a symmetrical rash over the extensor surfaces of the arms, legs and buttocks.

Questions

1. What is the likely diagnosis?
The likely diagnosis is Henoch–Schonlein purpura.

2. What is the underlying pathophysiology?
This is thought to be due to increased circulating IgA levels and disruption of IgG synthesis. These interact to produce complexes that activate the complement system, leading to vasculitis.

3. What other symptoms can a child present with?
Children can also present with joint pain and glomerulonephritis (e.g. haematuria, oliguria). Intussusception can be a presenting complication.

4. For how long should a child be followed up?
Any child who has renal involvement should be followed up for 1 year to detect those who have persisting problems and who therefore require longer term follow-up.

A 5-year-old girl attends the emergency department with an exacerbation of her asthma. She was noted to have an itchy rash affecting the antecubital fossae.

Questions

1. What is the likely diagnosis?
The likely diagnosis is atopic eczema.

2. What is the management?
Atopic eczema is managed by avoiding irritants such as biological washing powder and soaps. Cotton clothes cause less irritation. Children's nails should be cut short to minimize skin damage. Emollients are the most important therapy. These should be applied two to three times a day. These include 50/50 (white soft paraffin/liquid paraffin) or aqueous cream. Topical corticosteroids should be used twice daily and the strength can be increased depending on treatment response. H1 histamine antagonists can be used to reduce itchiness. Bandages may be helpful if there is widespread eczema in young children. In children over 2 years, tacrolimus can be used topically to reduce the use of topical corticosteroids.

3. At what age would you expect this condition to have resolved by?
Atopic eczema resolves by 12 years in 50% of children and by 16 years in 75% of children.

4. List some differentials of an itchy rash.
Causes of an itchy rash include fungal infections, scabies, chicken pox, urticaria and insect bites.

3: Psychiatry

GENERAL PSYCHIATRIC HISTORY

When taking a history, it is important to try to develop good rapport with the patient. This is particularly true for the psychiatric history. Although it is useful to be systematic in your questioning, the patient may initially not feel comfortable answering some of the more personal questions and so flexibility is required. More personal questions can be returned to later in the interview if necessary.

'Mrs A attends the general psychiatry outpatient clinic complaining of low mood. Please take a general psychiatric history.'

Score Sheet

Scores: 1 = Not attempted; 2 = Attempted, unsatisfactory; 3 = Attempted, satisfactory

Action	1	2	3
Introduction			
1. Check the patient's name, age, marital status and occupation			
Presenting complaint			
2. What is the patient's current problem (in their own words or paraphrase) and for how long has it been an issue?			
History of presenting complaint			
3. Explore the patient's main symptom in detail: onset, progression, severity (functional impact), alleviating/aggravating factors			
4. Explore associated physical/biological, psychological and social features			
5. What treatments has the patient tried already?			
Past psychiatric history			
6. Any previous psychiatric problems (diagnosed or non-diagnosed)?			
7. Any history of self-harm?			
Past medical history			
8. Any previous medical problems?			
Drug history			
9. Any prescribed, alternative or over-the-counter medications? Any recent change?			
10. Any adverse reactions to medications?			

Continued

Action	1	2	3
Family history			
11. Ascertain a family tree, including significant illness, and explore family relationships			
Social history			
12. Current circumstances: accommodation, financial situation, hobbies, family/social support			
13. Smoking, alcohol and recreational drug history (detailed)			
14. Forensic history (arrest/convictions)			
Personal history			
15. Explore patient's childhood, educational achievements, occupational history, psychosexual history, traumatic events and religious orientations			
Pre-morbid personality			
16. Elicit how the patient would describe his or her normal self before he or she began experiencing current problems			
Ideas/concerns/expectations			
17. Explore the patient's ideas/concerns/expectations			
Summary			
18. Summarize the findings to the patient, clarifying any errors. Thank the patient and present findings to the examiner			
Overall score		/54	

1. **Name/age/marital status/occupation.** These are important factors to ascertain in all patients. They not only help to ensure correct identity but can also impact on prognosis and treatment.
2. **Current problem.** Many patients are referred by another clinician, in which case the reason for their presentation should be in the referral letter. Nonetheless, it is important to ascertain from patients what they consider the main issue to be and for how long they consider that it has been a problem.
3. **History of problem.** Explore in depth how the patient's issues have progressed over time and what impact his or her problems are having on their quality of life and functional ability.
4. **Associated features.** Many mental health problems have physical effects (e.g. poor sleep, poor appetite) and social effects (e.g. social anxiety, social withdrawal), and it is important to enquire about these.
5. **Treatments tried.** Many patients will have tried treatments already (prescribed or non-prescribed), and you should determine what these were and what effect they had.
6. **Previous psychiatric problems.** Determine whether the patient has had any mental health problems diagnosed in the past. Also enquire about any problems that were not brought to medical attention.

7. **History of self-harm.** This is an important part of the risk assessment.
8. **Previous medical problems.** A past medical history is just as important in a psychiatric history as in a medical history. Certain medical problems may predispose to mental health problems and can also have an impact on treatment options.
9. **Medications.** Find out what medications the patient is taking (prescribed, over the counter) and whether there has been any recent change in medication. If there has been a recent change, find out if this has had any effect on his or her current problems.
10. **Adverse reactions to medications.** This is important to ask in any history as it can affect treatment options.
11. **Family tree.** It is often helpful to try and draw a family tree as family connections and significant illnesses (medical and psychiatric) may be important. Try to ascertain the quality of the relationships and whether there have been any recent major events in the family.
12. **Current circumstances.** Try to build a picture of the patient's current social situation by enquiring about his or her current accommodation, financial situation, hobbies and support network.
13. **Smoking, alcohol, recreational drugs.** The drug and alcohol history should be detailed. If there is a history of substance misuse, find out which substances the patient uses and the age at which this began. Explore whether there is any evidence of dependence (e.g. craving, tolerance, withdrawal effects) and whether the patient ever sought help for their problems. Ask about their pattern of alcohol intake (e.g. binge drinking, social drinking, daytime drinking).
14. **Forensic history.** Ask whether the patient ever had any problems with law enforcement agencies. If so, could these problems be related to any previous episodes of mental illness?
15. **Personal history.** This is a large and important part of the psychiatric history as it can sometimes provide useful clues to the patient's current problems. The personal history should include:
    a. **Childhood events:** Emotional problems, serious illnesses, bullying
    b. **Educational achievements:** Academic record, experience at school, friends at school
    c. **Occupational history:** Jobs in chronological order, job satisfaction, reason for job change
    d. **Psychosexual history:** Relationship history, quality of relationships, sexual problems
    e. **Traumatic events:** Any previous abuse or assaults
    f. **Religious orientations:** Any religious/spiritual beliefs
16. **Pre-morbid personality.** Ask when the patient last felt mentally and physically well. Find out what their personality used to be like, including predominant mood, sociability, motivation, hobbies and beliefs. It can also be helpful to ask how others would have described the patient's personality before he or she became unwell.

17. **Ideas, concerns, expectations.** Ask if the patient has any particular concerns or expectations or any questions.
18. **Summary.** All histories should be completed by clarifying the pertinent points of the history with the patient, thanking the patient and presenting a summary of your findings to the examiner.

MENTAL STATE EXAMINATION

The mental state examination is a structured way of assessing the patient's mental state at that moment in time. It includes subjective and objective information, and in combination with the information obtained from the general psychiatric history, it helps with the formulation of a clinical diagnosis and risk assessment.

'You have now taken a general psychiatric history from Mrs A. Please perform a mental state examination. Note, you are not required to perform a mini mental state examination.'

Score Sheet

Scores: 1 = Not attempted; 2 = Attempted, unsatisfactory; 3 = Attempted, satisfactory

Action	1	2	3
Appearance and behaviour			
1. *Appearance:* dress, self-care, unusual items carried, physical health (e.g. body mass index [BMI]), self-harm			
2. *Behaviour:* eye contact, facial expressions, rapport, activity, abnormal posture/gait			
Mood			
3. Subjective mood (the patient's report) and objective mood (the examiner's impression)			
4. Ideas of self-harm/suicide			
Speech			
5. Characteristics of speech			
6. Form of speech			
Thoughts			
7. Form of thought (how thoughts are expressed)			
8. Content of thought (what thoughts are expressed): preoccupations, abnormal beliefs, obsessions/compulsions			
9. Ideas of harm to others			
Perceptions			
10. Hallucinations, illusions, distortions, imagery			

Continued

Action	1	2	3
Cognitive state			
11. Is the patient oriented in time, place and person?			
12. Any memory problems?			
Insight			
13. Explore the patient's understanding of his or her condition and need for treatment			
Summary			
14. Summarize findings to the examiner			
Overall score		/42	

1. **Appearance.** Note whether the patient is appropriately dressed, his or her physical health (e.g. apparent BMI) and degree of self-care. Be alert to signs of self-harm or intravenous drug use (e.g. scars).
2. **Behaviour.** Does the patient make appropriate eye contact and is there good rapport? Are the patient's posture, body language and facial expressions appropriate?
3. **Subjective and objective mood.** Ask the patient to describe his or her mood (subjective mood) and also make a judgement yourself on what you consider the patient's mood to be (objective mood). Is the mood labile, reactive or flat and is it congruent with the content of their speech (i.e. is it appropriate for what the patient is talking about)? Also ask about anxiety symptoms.
4. **Ideas of self-harm.** This can be a difficult topic to broach. It sometimes helps to normalize the question, for example, 'Sometimes people with similar problems to yours have thoughts of harming themselves or feel that life is no longer worth living. Do you ever feel like that?'
5. **Speech characteristics.** Note the amount, rate, volume, fluency and tone of speech.

Disorders of speech ability

Dysphasia	Impairment of ability to express (expressive dysphasia) or comprehend (receptive dysphasia) speech
Dysarthria	Impairment of ability to articulate phonemes/words
Dysphonia	Impairment of ability to produce voice sounds

Disorders of rate and amount of speech

Pressure of speech	Increased rate and quantity of speech
Logorrhoea	Increased quantity of speech
Poverty of speech	Decreased quantity of speech
Psychomotor retardation	Decreased rate of speech (as well as other effects)

6. **Form of speech.** Note any abnormalities in the form of their speech.

Disorders of form of speech

Circumstantiality	Speech contains unnecessary detail, resulting in a delay in getting to the point
Tangentiality	Speech contains irrelevant replies and never gets to the point
Echolalia	Immediate, involuntary repetition of words/phrases spoken by others
Coprolalia	Involuntary expression of obscene language (a complex vocal tic)
Neologism	Use of a new word whose meaning is only known to the patient
Clang association	Linkage of words based on sound rather than meaning
Word salad	Meaningless mixture of words and phrases

7. **Form of thought.** The form of thought refers to **how** the thoughts are expressed and can be assessed by noting the way in which the patient responds to a question and whether you can follow their train of thought.

Disorders of form of thought

Flight of ideas	Rapid flow of accelerated speech in which the patient abruptly changes from one topic to another, usually with discernible associations
Loosening of associations	Ideas appear to shift from one topic to another but in an unrelated manner
Perseveration	Inappropriate persistence or repetition of a thought
Thought block	Interruption of a train of thought

8. **Content of thought.** The content of thought refers to **what** thoughts are expressed. Enquire about preoccupations, morbid thoughts, abnormal beliefs and obsessions/compulsions:
   a. **Preoccupations:** Does the patient spend excess time thinking about a particular subject?
   b. **Morbid thoughts:** Does the patient have thoughts of suicide, harming others, low self-esteem, guilt?
   c. **Abnormal beliefs:**
      i. **Delusions:** Fixed beliefs that are held with strong conviction in spite of insufficient evidence and that are not held by other people from the individual's background culture, e.g. paranoid delusions (persecutory, guilt, jealousy etc.), nihilistic delusions, delusions of control.

Delusions of control

Thought insertion	The belief that thoughts are being inserted into their mind by an external source
Thought withdrawal	The belief that their thoughts are being taken from their head by an external source

Continued

Delusions of control

Thought broadcasting	The belief that their thoughts are being made available to other people
Somatic passivity	The belief that bodily sensations are being received from an external source

     ii. **Overvalued ideas:** Unreasonable and sustained preoccupation with a belief that is not quite delusional in intensity (e.g. overvalued idea regarding body size in anorexia nervosa).

   d. **Obsessions/compulsions:** An obsession is a persistent preoccupation with an often-unwanted idea. A compulsion refers to a behaviour that a person feels compelled to perform in response to an obsession. It is important to try to determine the fear underlying the obsession and elucidate the impact of the obsession on daily life.

9. **Ideas of harming others.** This can also be a difficult topic to broach but is important with regard to risk assessment.

10. **Perceptions.** Abnormal perceptions generally refer to hallucinations, illusions and distortions.

   a. **Hallucinations:** The perception of visual, auditory, olfactory, gustatory or tactile experiences without an external stimulus.

   b. **Illusions:** A false perception of a real external stimulus.

   c. **Distortions:** Could refer to a distortion of the patient's sense of time, memory or place (e.g. déjà vu), distortion in the patient's awareness of the external world (derealization) or distortion in sense of self (depersonalization).

   d. **Imagery:** Mental images/pictures that may be distressing to the individual, for example, in post-traumatic stress disorder (PTSD).

11. **Oriented in time, place and person.** Ascertain whether the patient is oriented in time, place and person and also note his or her attention and concentration ability. Concentration can be assessed with the serial sevens test (ask the patient to count down from 100 in sevens).

12. **Memory problems.** If you suspect memory problems, there are a variety of formal tests that you can perform, e.g. mini mental state examination (MMSE) and Hopkins Verbal Learning Test (HVLT).

13. **Insight.** Insight refers to the patient's understanding of his or her condition and whether the patient recognizes his or her need for treatment. This can fluctuate over time.

14. **Summary.** Summarize your findings to the examiner and offer a differential diagnosis, if possible.

Clinical scenario: schizophrenia

Vignette

Mr A is a 19-year-old student who has been brought to A&E by his mother due to her concern at his increasingly bizarre behaviour. Take a history and assess his mental state.

Presentation

Mr A is a 19-year-old student who has been brought to hospital by his concerned mother. For the past 3 months, he has been spending a significant amount of time in his room and has reported that he can hear the neighbours talking about him and plotting to kill him. He has been experiencing poor sleep and has fallen behind with his studies and stopped going out with friends. Until now he has refused medical help and so has not received any treatment to date. There is no previous history of medical or psychiatric problems, and he takes no medications. He has an uncle who suffers from schizophrenia, and his mother had postnatal depression. Mr A lives with his parents and smokes 15 cigarettes per day. He smoked cannabis between the ages of 14 and 17. He has never been in trouble with the police. He has only had one short-lived relationship. Mr A describes himself as having been a shy child with not many friends.

On mental state examination, Mr A appeared unkempt and underweight. He had poor eye contact, and it was difficult to establish rapport. He reported his mood as good but objectively his mood appeared flat. He denied any thoughts of self-harm or thoughts of harming other people. He had poverty of speech with some tangentiality. There was evidence of loosening of associations and occasional thought block. He reported that his thoughts were preoccupied with his neighbours, and he believed that they were withdrawing thoughts from his head (thought withdrawal). At several points, he appeared to be responding to external stimuli and reported third-person auditory hallucinations. He was oriented in time, place and person and did not appear to have any memory problems. He understands that he is unwell but attributes his problems to his persecution by his neighbours. He lacks full insight into his current difficulties.

Based on my assessment, Mr A's presentation would fit with a diagnosis of psychosis.

Questions

1. In a patient with psychotic symptoms, what could be the differential diagnosis?

The causes of psychosis can be divided into psychiatric disorders and medical disorders. Examples of each are shown in the table below.

Psychiatric disorders	Medical disorders
Schizophrenia	Epilepsy
Schizotypal disorder	Space-occupying lesion
Schizoaffective disorder	CNS infections
Psychotic depression	Dementia

Continued

Psychiatric disorders	Medical disorders
Delusional disorders	Huntington's disease
Manic episode	Wilson disease
Drug-induced psychosis	Porphyria
Puerperal psychosis	Systemic lupus erythematosus (SLE)

2. What further assessment would you undertake in a patient with psychosis (after history and mental state examination)?

Further assessment of a patient with psychosis would involve a full physical examination, blood tests (to include FBC, U&Es, LFTs, TFTs, glucose, lipids, ESR), urinalysis and drug screen. An ECG should be recorded before commencing pharmacological treatment, and a head CT and EEG may also be warranted (for example, if there is concern about temporal lobe epilepsy or intracranial mass).

3. How common is schizophrenia and at what age does it typically present?

Schizophrenia has a prevalence of approximately 1% and affects males and females equally. It can present at any age but is uncommon after age 45. The mean age of onset in males is 28 and in females is 32. The onset of schizophrenia is often preceded by a prodromal phase that can last for several years. This prodromal phase generally involves a subtle decline in cognitive ability and behaviour.

4. What are Schneider's first-rank symptoms?

In the 1950s, a psychiatrist named Kurt Schneider listed specific psychotic symptoms that he believed distinguished schizophrenia from other psychotic disorders (see the following table). These are called 'first-rank symptoms'. However, although they contribute to the current diagnostic criteria for schizophrenia, they are also found in other psychotic disorders and are absent in up to 20% of patients with schizophrenia.

Schneider's first-rank symptoms

Auditory hallucinations

Audible thoughts	Thoughts are 'heard' (thought echo)
Third person	Voices discuss or argue about the patient
Running commentary	Voices comment on the patient's behaviour, thoughts and actions

Delusions of thought control

Thought withdrawal	Thoughts are being removed from the patient's mind by an external source
Thought insertion	Thoughts are being put into the patient's mind by an external source
Thought broadcasting	The patient's thoughts are accessible to others

Continued

Schneider's first-rank symptoms

Delusions of passivity

'Made' volition	The patient's volitions are under control of an external source
'Made' affects, feelings or impulses	The patient's emotions and impulses are under control of an external source
Somatic passivity	The patient's bodily sensations are under the control of an external source
Delusional perception	A normal perception is interpreted in a delusional way

5. What risk factors for schizophrenia have been identified?

Numerous biological, psychological and social risk factors that are believed to predispose, precipitate and perpetuate schizophrenia have been identified. Examples are found in the following table.

	Biological	Psychological	Social
Predisposing factors	Genetic factors Obstetric complications Season of birth (higher relative risk in those born in the winter months)		Lower socioeconomic class Immigration
Precipitating factors	Illicit drugs (e.g. cannabis, cocaine, Ecstasy)	Adverse life events/ stress	Immigration to a developed country
Perpetuating factors	Ongoing cannabis use	Exposure to high expressed emotion in a close relative (>35 hours/week)	Ongoing social stress

6. What are the treatment options for schizophrenia?

Immediate management options would involve deciding whether the patient needs inpatient treatment or whether the patient could be managed as an outpatient. Treatment options can then be divided into biological, psychological and social treatments and often a combination of approaches is used.

Biological	Psychological	Social
• Antipsychotics • First line = atypical • Second line = different class • Third line = clozapine • Other medications (e.g. lithium, benzodiazepine) • Electro-convulsive therapy (ECT)	• Psychoeducation • Family education • Cognitive behavioural therapy (CBT), especially for any residual psychotic symptoms	• Self-help groups • Rehabilitation (consider involvement of occupational therapist [OT]) • Involvement of community psychiatric nurse (CPN) • Social skills training

7. **What is this patient's prognosis?**
As a general rule, after the first acute psychotic episode, one-third of patients will recover completely, one-third will improve but continue to experience significant symptoms and one-third will not improve and will require frequent hospitalization for their symptoms. Approximately 10% will commit suicide in the first 5 years after diagnosis. Factors associated with a poorer prognosis include insidious onset, young age at onset (under 25), male sex, substance misuse, early negative symptoms (such as poverty of speech, apathy and social withdrawal) and non-compliance with medication.

8. **What is neuroleptic malignant syndrome?**
Neuroleptic malignant syndrome is a rare but potentially fatal reaction to neuroleptic or antipsychotic medications. It is thought to be caused by central dopamine D_2 receptor blockade or dopamine depletion and is characterized by muscle rigidity, hyperthermia, autonomic instability and altered mental status. It can lead to rhabdomyolysis, seizures, arrhythmias and death. Treatment involves stopping the offending drug and supportive treatment (IV fluids, cooling blankets). Dantrolene – a muscle relaxant – may be used to reduce muscle rigidity.

CLINICAL SCENARIO: ASSESSMENT OF DEPRESSION

Depression is common and affects people in many different ways, causing a wide variety of symptoms. The '2-Question screening test' can be used as a quick tool to identify patients who may be having problems with low mood. If they score positively on this, a more detailed depression assessment is warranted. This would involve a full psychiatric history and mental state examination but with the addition of questions that specifically explore depressive symptoms in depth. In an OSCE, you may be asked to perform a full psychiatric assessment or you may be asked to just focus on the depressive symptoms.

2-Question screening test
Score Sheet

Scores: 1 = Not attempted; 2 = Attempted, unsatisfactory; 3 = Attempted, satisfactory

Action	1	2	3
1. During the past month, have you often been bothered by feeling down, depressed or hopeless?			
2. During the past month, have you been bothered by little interest or pleasure in doing things?			
3. (If answer to question 2 is positive) Do you want help for these problems?			
Overall score		/9	

Depression assessment

Score Sheet

Scores: 1 = Not attempted; 2 = Attempted, unsatisfactory; 3 = Attempted, satisfactory

Action	1	2	3
1. Ask how their mood has been recently and how often they feel like that			
2. Have they lost interest in their usual activities?			
3. Have they noticed a decrease in their energy levels?			
4. Have they been feeling restless or been moving around more than usual?			
5. Have they been feeling slowed down as though they were moving slowly?			
6. How has their sleep been? How does this compare to before?			
7. Has there been any change in their appetite or weight?			
8. How has their ability to concentrate been?			
9. Have they been experiencing feelings of guilt or been blaming themselves for things?			
10. Any suicidal ideation or thoughts of harming themselves?			
Overall score		/30	

Case 1: depression

Vignette

Mrs D is a 32-year-old housewife who has been referred by her GP with low mood. Please enquire further about her recent mood problems.

Presentation

Mrs D is a 32-year-old housewife who has been referred by her GP for assessment. For the past 6 months, she has been feeling low in mood every day, worse in the mornings. She used to enjoy gardening and shopping but has found that she has lost interest in these activities. She feels lethargic most days, which she attributes to poor sleep, with early morning waking. Her appetite is reduced, but she has not lost any weight. She used to be able to concentrate on reading a book but finds that she now struggles to read one page. She denies any feelings of guilt but admits to occasional thoughts of self-harm.

Based on my assessment, Mrs D's presentation would fit with a diagnosis of depressive disorder.

Questions

1. What further assessment would you undertake in this patient?
   Further assessment of this patient would involve a full psychiatric history, including past medical history and medication history. It would also be important to perform a full physical examination and blood tests

(to include FBC, U&Es, LFTs, TFTs, vitamin B12, folate, ESR) to rule out possible physical causes of depression. A CT head may be warranted (if concerned about an intracranial mass). A mood diary would be helpful to gain better insight into the patient's current difficulties.

2. What is the differential diagnosis of depression?
The differential diagnoses of depression can be divided into psychiatric disorders and medical disorders. Examples of each are shown in the table below.

Psychiatric disorders	Medical disorders
Depressive episode	Neurological: Alzheimer, Huntingdon, multiple sclerosis
Recurrent depressive episode	Endocrine: Cushing, hypothyroidism, hyperparathyroidism
Bipolar affective disorder	Metabolic: anaemic, B12/folate deficiency, hypercalcaemia
Dysthymia	Infective: influenza, Epstein–Barr virus, HIV
Cyclothymia	Neoplastic: paraneoplastic syndrome
Mixed affective state	Drugs: steroids, non-steroidal anti-inflammatory drugs
Seasonal affective disorder	(NSAIDs), beta-blockers, L-Dopa
Schizoaffective disorder	Alcohol
Adjustment disorder	
Bereavement	

3. What risk factors for depression have been identified?
Numerous biological, psychological and social risk factors that are believed to predispose, precipitate and perpetuate depression have been identified. Examples of each are given below.

	Biological	Psychological	Social
Predisposing factors	Family history Female gender	Personality (neuroticism, obsessionality) Cluster C (anxious) personality disorders	Early adverse life events
Precipitating factors	Organic causes	Diagnosis of terminal illness	Adverse life events
Perpetuating factors	Substance misuse	Cognitive distortions	Social withdrawal

4. What are cognitive distortions?
Cognitive distortions are exaggerated and irrational thoughts that may perpetuate psychiatric disorders such as depression. They include:
a. Dichotomous thinking: all-or-nothing thinking
b. Overgeneralization: drawing a general conclusion based on a single incident
c. Magnification/minimization: over- or underestimating the importance of an event

d. Personalization: believing that everything that happens is a result of something they have done

e. Catastrophic thinking: always expecting disaster to strike

5. What are the clinical features of depression?

The clinical features found in depression can be categorized into biological, psychological and social features.

Biological	Psychological	Social
Weight loss/gain	Low mood	Reduced social interaction
Appetite change	Anhedonia	Work absences
Sleep disturbance	Reduced concentration	Decreased hobbies
Early morning waking	Feelings of guilt	
Fatigue	Poor self-esteem	
Constipation	Pessimism	
Reduced libido	Ideas of deliberate	
Agitation/retardation	self-harm/suicide	
	Hopelessness	

6. What are the treatment options for depression?

Immediate management options would involve deciding whether the patient needs inpatient treatment or whether they could be managed as an outpatient. Treatment options can then be divided into biological, psychological and social treatments, and often a combination of approaches is used.

Biological	Psychological	Social
• Antidepressants	• Psychoeducation	• Exercise/new hobbies
• Augmentation of antidepressants with other drugs (e.g. low-dose second-generation antipsychotic, lithium, or triiodothyronine)	• Cognitive behavioural therapy (CBT)	• Sleep hygiene
	• Psychotherapy	• Befriending scheme
	• Counselling	• Involvement of community psychiatric nurse (CPN)
• ECT	• Self-help	
• Abstain from alcohol		

7. What is this patient's prognosis?

After the first depressive episode, approximately 80% of patients have a further depressive episode; subsequent episodes tend to become progressively longer and the interval between episodes becomes shorter. Ten per cent develop a chronic disorder and 10% develop a manic episode (and so are diagnosed with bipolar affective disorder). Seven per cent of males and 1% of females with severe depression commit suicide.

CLINICAL SCENARIO: ASSESSMENT OF MANIA

Although mania is usually considered in the context of bipolar disorder, it is important to remember that mania can be a feature of other psychiatric disorders, such as schizoaffective disorder. Assessment of a patient with mania would involve a full psychiatric history and mental state examination but with the addition of questions that specifically explore mania symptoms in depth. In an OSCE, you may be asked to perform a full psychiatric assessment, or you may be asked to just focus on the mania symptoms.

Score Sheet

Scores: 1 = Not attempted; 2 = Attempted, unsatisfactory; 3 = Attempted, satisfactory

Action	1	2	3
1. Have they felt their mood is so elevated that other people felt they were not themselves?			
2. Have they felt more self-confident than normal?			
3. Have they been feeling restless or been moving around more than usual?			
4. Have they found they need less sleep than normal?			
5. Have they felt more irritable than normal or been involved in more arguments than normal?			
6. Have they been more talkative than normal?			
7. Have they felt that their thoughts were racing?			
8. How has their concentration been?			
9. How have their energy levels been?			
10. Have they been more sociable than normal?			
11. Have they been engaging in activities that other people have considered foolish or risky?			
12. Have they been spending more money than normal?			
13. As a result of the above, have they had any problems with money, legal troubles, family or work?			
Overall score		/39	

Case 1: mania

Vignette

Ms M is a 26-year-old secretary who has been brought for review by a friend who is concerned about her recent behaviour with elevated mood and reckless spending. Please assess her for a possible diagnosis of mania.

Presentation

Ms M is a 26-year-old secretary who has been brought for review by her friend who is concerned about her mental health. For the past 2 weeks, Ms M has felt that her mood and self-confidence have been significantly elevated compared to normal. She has been persistently restless and is only sleeping for around 2 hours per night. Ms M believes her concentration and energy levels have been elevated, and she finds that her thoughts race through her head. Her friend reports that she sometimes speaks so fast that it is difficult to understand what she is saying. Ms M has recently become much more sociable but has started getting into fights, which her friend reports is out of character for her. She recently spent £20,000 on a new car and, despite previously being scared of heights, has booked a sky-diving holiday in South America. She has fallen out with her family and is in trouble with her bank.

Based on my assessment, Ms M's presentation would fit with a diagnosis of mania.

Questions

1. What further assessment would you undertake in this patient?

   Further assessment of this patient would involve a full psychiatric history, including past medical history and medication history. It would also be important to perform a full physical examination, blood tests (to include FBC, U&Es, LFTs, TFTs, vitamin B12, folate, ESR) and drug screen. An ECG should be recorded before commencing pharmacological treatment, and a CT head may be warranted (if concerned about an intracranial mass). A mood diary would be helpful to gain a better insight into the patient's current difficulties. (Notice that this answer is the same as that given for depression. It would be useful to memorize something similar to this as a 'stock' answer.)

2. What is the differential diagnosis of mania?

   The differential diagnoses of mania can be divided into psychiatric disorders and medical disorders. Examples of each are shown in the following table.

Psychiatric disorders	Medical disorders
Bipolar affective disorder	Frontal lobe disorder: stroke,
Cyclothymia	multiple sclerosis, intracranial
Mixed affective state	mass, epilepsy
Schizophrenia	Cushing syndrome
Schizoaffective disorder	Hyperthyroidism
Substance misuse	Systemic lupus erythematosus
Attention-deficit hyperactivity	Sleep deprivation
disorder (ADHD)	

3. What is the difference between mania and hypomania?

   The clinical features of mania and hypomania are very similar; however, in hypomania, there are no psychotic features and there is no impairment in social functioning.

4. What risk factors for bipolar disorder have been identified?

   Numerous biological, psychological and social risk factors that are believed to predispose, precipitate and perpetuate bipolar affective disorder have been identified. Examples are given in the following table.

	Biological	Psychological	Social
Predisposing factors	Family history		Higher socioeconomic class
Precipitating factors	Sleep disturbance Early postpartum period	Severe stresses	Adverse life events Late spring/summer
Perpetuating factors	Sleep disturbance Substance misuse Non-compliance with medications		

5. What are the treatment options for bipolar affective disorder?
Immediate management options would involve deciding whether the patient needs inpatient treatment or whether they could be managed as an outpatient. Treatment options can then be divided into biological, psychological and social treatments and often a combination of approaches is used.

Biological	Psychological	Social
Acute mania: • Stop antidepressants • Antipsychotics • Benzodiazepines • Mood stabilizers • ECT if refractory to medication Maintenance: • Mood stabilizers	• Psychoeducation (e.g. relapse prevention) • Self-help groups • Cognitive behavioural therapy (CBT)	• Avoid relapse triggers • Sleep hygiene • Involvement of community psychiatric nurse (CPN)

6. What is the prognosis for this patient?
After the first manic episode, approximately 90% of patients have further manic and/or depressive episodes, and the interval between each episode tends to become shorter. Approximately 10% of patients commit suicide. Concordance with medication and avoidance of substance misuse are key factors in prognosis.

CLINICAL SCENARIO: ASSESSMENT OF ANXIETY

Anxiety symptoms can be found in coexistence with other psychiatric illnesses, or they may be significant enough to be classified as a disorder in their own right. Assessment of a patient with anxiety would involve a full psychiatric history and mental state examination but with the addition of questions that specifically explore anxiety symptoms in depth. In an OSCE, you may be asked to perform a full psychiatric assessment, or you may be asked to just focus on the anxiety symptoms.

Score Sheet

Scores: 1 = Not attempted; 2 = Attempted, unsatisfactory; 3 = Attempted, satisfactory

Action	1	2	3
Elicitation of anxiety symptoms			
1. Ask them to describe their anxiety symptoms and for how long they have been a problem. Was there a triggering event?			
2. When they feel anxious do they have any associated physical symptoms?			
3. Do they ever have a sense of impending doom?			
Circumstances of anxiety symptoms			
4. Are the anxiety symptoms present all the time or just in certain circumstances/situations?			
5. Do they avoid certain circumstances/situations because they know these will trigger their symptoms?			
Other symptoms			
6. Do they ever find it difficult to relax or feel so restless that they are unable to sit still?			
7. Are they more irritable than they used to be?			
8. Do they find that they are unable to stop worrying about things?			
Depressive symptoms			
9. Any problems with low mood or somatic symptoms of depressive disorder (e.g. early morning waking, poor appetite etc.)?			
10. If they have problems with low mood, did this start before or after the anxiety problems?			
Impact of symptoms on life			
11. What impact are their symptoms having on their life?			
Overall score		/33	

Case 1: agoraphobia with panic attacks
Vignette

Mrs P is a 34-year-old homemaker who has been brought for assessment by her husband who is concerned that she is finding it increasingly difficult to leave the house due to anxiety. Please perform an assessment of her anxiety problems.

Presentation

Mrs P is a 34-year-old homemaker who has been brought for assessment by her concerned husband. Her symptoms started 6 months ago when she was in a supermarket and suddenly became sweaty, dizzy and anxious. She was terrified that she was going to die and felt everyone was staring at her. Since then she has been fearful of leaving the house and becomes anxious in crowded public places. On four separate occasions, these anxiety symptoms have been associated with palpitations, sweating, breathlessness and a sense of impending doom, fearing that she is going to die. She has been avoiding leaving the house due to fear that her symptoms will recur. She reports no anxiety when at home and denies any symptoms of restlessness, irritability or generalized worry. Over the past 2 months, she has started to feel low in mood due to the impact her anxiety symptoms are having on her life. She feels she can no longer safely leave her house, and so can no longer do the grocery shopping for her family or meet up with friends. Her problems are putting a strain on her marriage.

Based on my assessment, Mrs P's presentation would fit with a diagnosis of agoraphobia with panic attacks.

Questions

1. What is agoraphobia?

   Agoraphobia is a persistent irrational fear of places that are difficult to escape from, such as shops, crowded places or when travelling on trains, buses or planes. Panic disorder is a frequent feature of episodes, and avoidance of the phobic situation is often a prominent feature.

2. What are the treatment options for agoraphobia?

   Treatment options can then be divided into biological, psychological and social treatments, and often a combination of approaches is used.

Biological	Psychological	Social
• Antidepressants (selective serotonin reuptake inhibitors [SSRIs] are first line) • Benzodiazepines may be used in the short term but can be addictive • Avoid anxiety-inducing substances, e.g. caffeine	• Cognitive behavioural therapy (CBT) • Psychoeducation • Self-help groups/Web sites	• Involvement of community psychiatric nurse (CPN) in severe cases

3. What is this patient's prognosis?

   Relapse is unfortunately very common, and one in five patients will attempt suicide.

CLINICAL SCENARIO: ASSESSMENT OF EATING DISORDERS

The SCOFF questionnaire was devised by John Morgan in Leeds in 1999 and involves five screening questions that can help identify patients with possible eating disorders. It is not considered diagnostic, but a positive answer to two or more questions should raise suspicion of anorexia nervosa or bulimia, which would warrant further in-depth assessment.

Score Sheet

Scores: 1 = Not attempted; 2 = Attempted, unsatisfactory; 3 = Attempted, satisfactory

Action	1	2	3
1. Do you make yourself **S**ICK because you feel uncomfortably full?			
2. Do you worry that you have lost **C**ONTROL over how much you eat?			
3. Have you recently lost more than **O**NE stone in weight in a 3-month period?			
4. Do you believe yourself to be **F**AT when others say you are too thin?			
5. Would you say **F**OOD dominates your life?			
Overall score		/15	

Case 1: anorexia nervosa

Vignette

Ms A is a 16-year-old student who has been brought for review by her mother who is concerned about her recent significant weight loss. Please assess whether she may be suffering from an eating disorder.

Presentation

Ms A is a 16-year-old student who has been brought for review by her mother. She has lost 2 stone in weight in the past 3 months. She denies self-induced vomiting but admits to worrying that she has lost control over how much she eats. She believes herself to be overweight despite other people telling her she appears too thin. She spends most of her day thinking about food.

Based on these questions, I believe that Ms A may be suffering from an eating disorder.

Questions

1. What further assessment would you undertake in this patient?

   Further assessment of this patient would involve a more detailed assessment of other symptoms of anorexia nervosa (e.g. using the EAT-26 [eating attitudes test questionnaire]), a full psychiatric history, including past medical history and medication history. It would also be important to perform a full physical examination (including BMI), blood tests (to include FBC, U&Es, LFTs, TFTs, calcium, magnesium, phosphate, glucose, serum iron) and an ECG. A food diary would be helpful to gain a better insight into the patient's eating habits.

2. What are the diagnostic criteria for anorexia nervosa?

   The diagnostic criteria for anorexia nervosa include:
   a. Body weight less than 85% of that expected for age and height
   b. Intense fear of gaining weight or becoming fat
   c. Disturbance in body image perception
   d. Amenorrhea (i.e. absence of at least three consecutive menstrual cycles)

3. What risk factors for anorexia nervosa have been identified?

Numerous biological, psychological and social risk factors that are believed to predispose, precipitate and perpetuate anorexia have been identified. These can be categorized as shown in the following table.

	Biological	Psychological	Social
Predisposing factors	Family history of eating disorder, mood disorder or substance abuse Female gender	Poor self-esteem Premorbid anxiety and depression Cluster C (anxious) personality disorders	Society pressures Family pressures (overprotection, rigidity)
Precipitating factors		Poor self-esteem Altered perception of body image	Life stressors, e.g. failing exam, moving school Bullying about weight
Perpetuating factors	Low body weight	Poor self-esteem Altered perception of body image	Society pressures Family pressures (overprotection, rigidity)

4. What are the treatment options for anorexia nervosa?

Immediate management options would involve deciding whether the patient needs inpatient treatment or whether they could be managed as an outpatient or day-patient. Treatment options can then be divided into biological, psychological and social treatments, and often a combination of approaches is used.

Biological	Psychological	Social
• Weight gain • May need inpatient medical treatment if physically unstable • Multivitamins	• Psychoeducation • Cognitive behavioural therapy (CBT) • Family therapy • Self-help groups	• Limit excessive exercise • Involvement of community psychiatric nurse (CPN)

5. What is this patient's prognosis?

As a general rule, if patients with anorexia nervosa receive treatment, one-third will make a complete recovery, one-third will partially recover and one-third will have chronic problems. The mortality for anorexia nervosa is the highest of any psychiatric illness at 15%–20%. Most deaths result from medical complications or suicide. Good prognostic factors include early age of onset, early treatment and good support network. Poor prognostic factors include long duration of illness, bulimic features, male gender and excessive weight loss.

CLINICAL SCENARIO: ASSESSMENT OF ALCOHOL DEPENDENCE

Alcohol dependence is often under-diagnosed in patients with mental health problems. The CAGE screening questionnaire can be used as a quick screening tool to identify patients that may be having problems with alcohol. If they score positively on this, then a more detailed alcohol assessment is warranted. This would involve a full psychiatric history and mental state examination but with the addition of questions that specifically explore alcohol dependence symptoms in depth. In an OSCE, you may be asked to perform a full psychiatric assessment, or you may be asked to just focus on the symptoms of alcohol dependence.

CAGE screening questionnaire

Score Sheet

Scores: 1 = Not attempted; 2 = Attempted, unsatisfactory; 3 = Attempted, satisfactory

Action	1	2	3
1. Have you ever felt that you should **C**ut down on your drinking?			
2. Have people **A**nnoyed you by criticizing your drinking?			
3. Have you ever felt bad or **G**uilty about drinking?			
4. Have you ever taken a drink first thing in the morning (**E**ye-opener)?			
Overall score		/12	

Two or more positive replies warrant a more detailed investigation into possible alcohol abuse.

Alcohol risk assessment/history

Score Sheet

Scores: 1 = Not attempted; 2 = Attempted, unsatisfactory; 3 = Attempted, satisfactory

Action	1	2	3
Introduction			
1. Explain that you are going to ask some questions about drinking habits and obtain consent.			
Alcohol intake			
2. Ask about amount and type of alcohol they drink (clarify the percentage alcohol in the drink).			
3. Ask about when and where they drink the alcohol. Do they always drink in the same place?			
Features of alcohol dependence			
4. Ask about compulsion to drink. Do they sometimes crave alcohol?			
5. Ask about primacy of drinking over other activities.			

Continued

Action	1	2	3
6. Ask about increased tolerance to alcohol. How much can they drink without feeling drunk and has this changed?			
7. Ask about withdrawal symptoms such as shaking, retching, sweating.			
8. Ask about relief drinking to avoid withdrawal symptoms (e.g. morning 'eye-opener').			
Psychiatric/medical history			
9. Any history of depression or other psychiatric illnesses?			
10. Any medical problems?			
Drug history			
11. Any prescribed, over-the-counter or recreational drugs?			
Social history			
12. Enquire about living conditions, employment, marital problems, financial problems.			
13. Forensic history (arrests/convictions).			
Questions/concerns			
14. Enquire whether the patient has any questions or concerns.			
Overall score		/42	

Case 1: alcohol use disorder
Vignette

Mr D is a 45-year-old accountant who has presented asking for help with excess alcohol intake, which he feels is affecting his functional ability. Please perform an alcohol assessment.

Presentation

Mr D is a 45-year-old accountant who has presented for help with his alcohol intake. For the past 8 months, he has been drinking up to one bottle of vodka per day. He used to just drink in the evenings at his local pub but is now drinking throughout the day in his own home. He feels a compulsion to drink as soon as he wakes up in the morning and, if he does not drink, he starts to feel unwell and shaky. He prioritizes buying alcohol over buying food and is finding that he needs more and more alcohol to prevent withdrawal symptoms. He has no history of psychiatric or medical problems and is on no regular medication. He was previously a high-functioning accountant but, in the past 8 months, he has missed a considerable amount of work and has been threatened with dismissal. He separated from his wife 2 months ago and is having financial problems. He has no forensic history.

Based on my assessment, Mr D appears to be suffering from alcohol use disorder.

Questions

1. What is the recommended daily limit for alcohol and what is the distinction between harmful and hazardous drinking?

   The recommended alcohol limit is 3–4 units per day for men (up to 21 per week) and 2–3 units per day for women (up to 14 per week). Harmful drinking refers to the intake of more than the recommended limit of alcohol in the absence of alcohol-related problems. Hazardous drinking refers to alcohol intake that is causing damage to the person's physical or mental health (excludes dependence).

2. What are the key features of alcohol use disorder (AUD)?

   According to the DSM-5 (*Diagnostic and Statistical Manual of Mental Disorders*, fifth edition), there are 11 key features of alcohol dependence. The presence of at least two of these suggests AUD:

   a. Alcohol is taken in larger amounts and over a longer period than intended

   b. There is a persistent desire or unsuccessful efforts to control alcohol use

   c. Much time is spent in activities necessary to obtain alcohol

   d. Existence of a craving to use alcohol

   e. Alcohol use results in a recurrent failure to fulfil major role obligations (work, school)

   f. There is continued use despite persistent social or interpersonal problems

   g. Important social/recreational activities are given up because of alcohol use

   h. There is recurrent alcohol use in situations where it is physically hazardous

   i. Use is continued despite knowledge of a persistent physical/psychological problem that is likely to be caused or exacerbated by alcohol

   j. Tolerance (increased amounts required for same effect, or diminished effects when drinking the same amount)

   k. Withdrawal (alcohol is taken to avoid withdrawal, or withdrawal symptoms are experienced)

3. What is delirium tremens?

   Delirium tremens is a potentially fatal condition that occurs in approximately 5% of alcohol-dependent patients 24–72 hours after stopping alcohol. It is a delirious condition characterized by confusion, agitation, clouding of/impaired consciousness, autonomic instability and perceptual disturbances. It can sometimes be associated with severe, uncontrollable tremors. Treatment involves benzodiazepines. The mortality rate can be as high as 35% if untreated but is less than 5% with treatment.

4. What is this patient's prognosis?

   Unfortunately, alcohol use disorder is a chronic relapsing condition, and only 20%–50% of patients remain abstinent 1 year after detoxification. Risk factors for relapse include lack of social support and comorbid psychiatric illness.

CLINICAL SCENARIO: ASSESSMENT OF SUICIDAL INTENT

Attempted suicide is a common presentation to the emergency department, and it is useful to be able to assess the degree of intent behind their attempt. The following questions are based on the Beck Suicide Intent Scale, which has high reliability and validity.

Score Sheet

Scores: 1 = Not attempted; 2 = Attempted, unsatisfactory; 3 = Attempted, satisfactory

Action	1	2	3
Objective circumstances related to suicide attempt			
1. Was anyone else present at the time?			
2. Did they make the attempt at a time when they thought someone would find them?			
3. Did they take any precautions against discovery/intervention and what were they?			
4. Did they make any arrangements in anticipation of death (e.g. will, gifts, insurance)?			
5. Was the attempt spontaneous or had they actively prepared for the attempt?			
6. Did they write a suicide note?			
7. Had they told anyone about their intentions prior to the attempt?			
8. Did they contact/notify anyone after the attempt?			
Self-report			
9. What was the purpose of their intent (e.g. to get attention, to get revenge, to escape, to surcease)?			
10. Did they think that their method would be lethal?			
11. Were they serious about ending their life?			
12. Did they want to die?			
13. Did they think that their death would be averted if they received medical attention?			
14. How long had they been thinking about suicide before the attempt?			
Other aspects			
15. How do they feel about the attempt now?			
16. Have they attempted suicide before?			
17. Had they been drinking alcohol or taken any recreational drugs at the time of the attempt?			
Overall score		/51	

Case 1: overdose

Vignette

Mrs O is a 40-year-old woman who was brought into A&E following an overdose of 30 citalopram tablets. She is medically fit for assessment. Please assess her suicide intent.

Presentation

Mrs O is a 40-year-old woman who was brought into A&E following an overdose of 30 citalopram with half a bottle of wine. She took the tablets at approximately 1 PM when she knew nobody would be home, and she closed the curtains so that no passerbys could see in. She had been preparing the attempt for approximately 1 week and had stockpiled tablets. She had written a suicide note but had not prepared her will. Nobody was aware of her intentions, and the only reason she was discovered was because her husband, who was meant to be at work all day, returned home unexpectedly, early in the afternoon. Mrs O states that her intent was to escape from her problems. She was certain that her method of choice would be lethal, even with delayed medical treatment (if she was found by her husband later that evening), as she was determined to die. Having survived the attempt, Mrs O still feels suicidal and thinks she will probably try to harm herself again.

Based on my assessment I believe that Mrs O displays signs of high suicide intent.

Questions

1. What are the risk factors for suicide?

   Risk factors for suicide can be divided into biological, psychological and social risk factors.

Biological	Psychological	Social
• Male sex (3 × more likely than women) • Age (male aged 25–44, female aged older than 65) • Chronic medical problems	• History of deliberate self-harm • Psychiatric disorder • Recent discharge from inpatient psychiatric care • Suicidal ideation • Depressed mood • Hopelessness • Impulsivity • Auditory hallucinations (especially commanding second person)	• Single, widowed, separated or divorced • Unemployed or retired • Certain occupations are higher risk: vets, doctors, pharmacists, farmers • Lower socioeconomic class • Poor level of social support • Recent life crisis

CLINICAL SCENARIO: ASSESSMENT OF CAPACITY

A person is assumed to have capacity unless it is established that they do not. The assessment of capacity can only be made about current capacity, not about past or future capacity, and it is specific to a particular decision. For example, they may have capacity to consent to give blood but not have capacity to refuse a life-saving operation. Capacity for each of these decisions must be assessed separately.

Score Sheet

Scores: 1 = Not attempted; 2 = Attempted, unsatisfactory; 3 = Attempted, satisfactory

Action	1	2	3
1. Can they understand the information relevant to the decision?			
2. Can they retain that information?			
3. Can they use or weigh that information as part of the process of making the decision?			
4. Can they communicate their decision (by talking, sign language or other means)?			
Overall score		/12	

A person is deemed to have capacity to make a particular decision only if they can fulfil all of the criteria above.

1. **Understand the information.** The information must be conveyed in a way that is appropriate to the patient's circumstances (e.g. using simple language or visual aids).
2. **Retain information.** Even if a person is only able to retain the information relevant to a decision for a short period, it does not prevent them from being regarded as able to make the decision.
3. **Weigh the information.** The information you provide should enable the patient to foresee the consequences of deciding one way or another or the consequences of failing to make the decision.
4. **Communicate the patient's decision.** This does not necessarily need to be verbal communication. It can be by sign language, writing or any other means possible.

Questions

1. What do you do if a patient lacks capacity?
   According to the Mental Capacity Act 2005, a person 'is not to be treated as unable to make a decision unless all practicable steps to help him to do so have been taken without success'. For example, if a patient lacks capacity because of delirium due to infection, if time permits (i.e. the decision to be made is not life threatening), steps should be taken to resolve the infection and then capacity can be reassessed. If the patient is still deemed to lack capacity, the professional must act in the patient's best interests. In this situation, the professional should consider the patient's past and present wishes and take into account the views of

carers/lasting power of attorney/deputy appointed by court as to what would be in the patient's best interests.

COMMUNICATION SKILLS

Commencing lithium therapy

Counselling a patient on commencing lithium therapy is a commonly encountered OSCE station because there is a range of information that must be covered, including side effects, need for monitoring and symptoms of toxicity to look out for.

Score Sheet

Scores: 1 = Does not perform well; 2 = Performs adequately; 3 = Performs well

Action	1	2	3
Introduction			
1. Greet the patient and introduce yourself (name and position).			
2. Confirm the patient's name and date of birth.			
3. Explain that you are going to talk to them about lithium therapy and establish what the patient already knows.			
What is lithium?			
4. Lithium is a mood stabilizer that helps to keep mood at a stable level, i.e. to prevent it going too high or going too low. The exact way in which lithium works is not known, but it appears to affect the transmission of important chemicals in the brain.			
What are the side effects?			
5. Immediate effects: side effects with lithium are, unfortunately, relatively common and include weight gain, tremor, tiredness, nausea, vomiting, acne, frequent urination, thirst and hair loss. Some of these side effects can be managed by altering the dose of lithium or by changing the lithium preparation. For many patients, however, there are no discernible adverse effects.			
6. Long-term side effects: in the long term, lithium can sometimes cause kidney changes and, rarely, may increase the risk of kidney failure (usually after at least 10 years of treatment). There is also the risk of developing an underactive thyroid (which can be treated with thyroid hormone replacement) and also a risk of hyperparathyroidism.			
7. If the (female) patient becomes pregnant while taking lithium, there is thought to be an increased risk of birth defects (in particular, congenital heart defects), although the balance of risks should be considered before lithium is stopped during pregnancy.			
Monitoring			
8. Before starting lithium, the patient will need a series of investigations, including blood tests (FBC, U&Es, TFTs, calcium), ECG and pregnancy test.			

Continued

Action	1	2	3
9. Regular blood monitoring is required to ensure that the levels of lithium in the blood are not too high, as this can be dangerous. Lithium levels will be checked 5 days after the first dose and then weekly until the lithium level is stable. It will then need to be tested every 3 months. Thyroid and kidney function will also be checked by a blood test every 6 months.			
10. It is important for the patient to be able recognize signs that the level of lithium in their blood may be becoming too high; these signs include blurred vision, coarse tremor, vomiting, diarrhoea, muscle weakness, unsteadiness and speech problems. If the patient experiences any of these, the patient should seek medical attention immediately.			
11. It is important that the patient maintains adequate fluid intake and avoids dietary changes that reduce or increase sodium levels because this can affect lithium levels.			
Finish			
12. Check that the patient understands what has been said.			
13. Ask if the patient has any questions.			
14. Offer a written information leaflet.			
Overall score	/42		

Questions

1. What conditions is lithium used for?

   Lithium is used for the treatment and prophylaxis of mania, bipolar disorder and recurrent depression.

2. What is the therapeutic range for lithium?

   The therapeutic range for lithium is 0.4–1.0 mmol/L.

Commencing SSRI antidepressant therapy

Counselling a patient on commencing antidepressant therapy is also a commonly encountered OSCE station. This station focuses on initiating SSRI (selective serotonin reuptake inhibitor) therapy, but you may also be asked to counsel the patient on the initiation of other antidepressants, e.g. tricyclic antidepressants or monoamine oxidase inhibitors.

Score Sheet

Scores: 1 = Does not perform well; 2 = Performs adequately; 3 = Performs well

Action	1	2	3
Introduction			
1. Greet the patient and introduce yourself (name and position).			
2. Confirm the patient's name and date of birth.			
3. Explain that you are going to talk to them about antidepressant therapy and establish what the patient already knows.			

Continued

Action	1	2	3
What is an antidepressant?			
4. An antidepressant is a medication commonly used in the treatment of mood disorders and anxiety. Their exact mechanism of action is unclear, but they are thought to work by affecting the balance of chemicals in the brain. In the case of SSRIs, they affect the balance of a chemical called serotonin.			
How long will it take to work?			
5. Most antidepressants take at least 2 weeks before they start to work, so the patient should not feel disheartened if they do not feel better straight away.			
What are the side effects of SSRIs?			
6. Immediate side effects include nausea, vomiting, indigestion, change in appetite and rash. They can occasionally affect the level of salts in the blood (hyponatraemia) and cause bleeding disorders.			
Duration of treatment/withdrawal			
7. To help prevent relapse, it is recommended that the antidepressant medication is continued for at least 6 months after the patient feels 'back to their normal self'.			
8. If the antidepressant is stopped abruptly, the patient may feel unwell (headaches, dizziness, shock-like sensations, change in mood), and it is often recommended that the dose is slowly tapered down. The patient should be advised to seek medical advice if they want to stop the medication.			
Finish			
9. Check that the patient understands what has been said.			
10. Ask if the patient has any questions.			
11. Offer a written information leaflet.			
Overall score		/33	

Questions

1. What would you advise if the patient became pregnant while taking an SSRI?

   As a general rule, SSRIs should be avoided in pregnancy unless the benefit outweighs the risk. If SSRIs are taken during early pregnancy, there may be an increase in risk of congenital heart disease. If they are taken in the third trimester, there may be a risk that when the baby is born it will experience withdrawal symptoms or persistent pulmonary hypertension.

2. What is serotonin syndrome?

   Serotonin syndrome is a rare but potentially fatal reaction caused by serotonergic medications, e.g. SSRIs, tricyclic antidepressants. It is characterized by a triad of cognitive effects (agitation, confusion, headache, hallucinations), autonomic effects (hyperthermia, shivering, hypertension, tachycardia, nausea) and somatic effects (tremor, myoclonus, hyperreflexia). It can lead to seizures and death. Treatment involves stopping the offending drug and starting supportive treatment (IV fluids, cooling blankets).

Explaining electro-convulsive therapy

A potential communication skills station in an OSCE could be explaining electro-convulsive therapy (ECT) to a patient. It is important to try to explain the procedure in simple terms and to leave time for the patient to ask any questions they may have.

Score Sheet

Scores: 1 = Does not perform well; 2 = Performs adequately; 3 = Performs well

Action	1	2	3
Introduction			
1. Greet the patient and introduce yourself (name and position).			
2. Confirm the patient's name and date of birth and the procedure that they are having.			
3. Ask if the patient has ever had ECT before and establish what they already know.			
The procedure			
4. Explain briefly what ECT is? ECT is a treatment used for a small number of patients with severe mental illnesses. It involves passing an electrical current through the brain in order to induce a fit. An anaesthetic and a muscle relaxant are given beforehand so that the patient is asleep when the current is given and the muscle spasms that would normally occur with a fit do not take place. Exactly how it works is still unknown, but it is believed that ECT causes a release of chemicals that help to improve conditions such as depression.			
Before the procedure			
5. Blood tests and an ECG are done before ECT treatment to make sure it is safe to have a general anaesthetic.			
6. The patient should not to eat or drink anything for 6 hours before the ECT (because of the anaesthetic).			
During the procedure			
7. Monitoring: the patient will be asked to lie on a trolley and will be connected to monitoring equipment to check pulse, blood pressure and oxygen levels. The patient will also be connected to an EEG machine to monitor their brain waves.			
8. Anaesthetic: the patient will be given a medicine through a needle (most likely in the back of the hand) to make them fall asleep.			
9. ECT: once the patient is asleep, a doctor will give the ECT treatment (the patient will remain asleep during this).			

Continued

Action	1	2	3
After the procedure			
10. On waking, the patient will be in a recovery room. The patient may feel a little nauseous to start with, but this should wear off within around 30 minutes.			
11. After recovery from the anaesthetic, the patient will be allowed to have some light refreshments and will then be allowed home/back to the ward. The whole process usually takes around 2 hours.			
Risks/side effects			
12. Short-term side effects include headache, muscle aching, muzzy-headedness. These often settle within a few hours with reassurance and simple painkillers. There may also be a temporary loss of memory.			
13. Long-term side effects include memory difficulties – most patients find this improves when the course of ECT has finished and a few weeks have passed. Some find it never recovers but it is unclear whether this is due to the ECT or to the depressive illness itself.			
Finish			
14. Check that the patient understands what has been said.			
15. Ask if the patient has any questions.			
16. Offer a written information leaflet.			
Overall score		/48	

Questions

1. What conditions is ECT used for?

   NICE guidelines recommend ECT for the treatment of symptoms of severe depressive illness, catatonia and prolonged or severe episodes of mania. It is only to be used if other treatments have failed or if the condition is potentially life threatening. ECT may be considered for patients with treatment-resistant schizophrenia in whom clozapine has been ineffective or not tolerated.

2. How many times is ECT given?

   ECT is often given twice a week and most patients receive a course of six to eight treatments. The patient should be reassessed after each ECT session, and there should be ongoing checks for any signs of memory loss.

3. Can ECT be given without consent?

   If a patient has capacity to consent but refuses, ECT may not be given, irrespective of their detention under the Mental Health Act. If the patient lacks capacity to consent and is not compliant with the treatment plan, a second opinion from a Second Opinion Appointed Doctor (SOAD) is needed before treatment can proceed. There is an exception, however, under Section 62 of the Act: if the psychiatrist deems the need for treatment is urgent, and they believe it is necessary to start ECT without authorization.

When a patient consents to ECT, written consent is obtained for a whole course of treatment and not just for each treatment session. It is important that the patient understand, however, that they can withdraw consent at any time, and the patient's verbal consent should be checked before each treatment session.

DATA INTERPRETATION

Clozapine monitoring

Clozapine can occasionally cause neutropenia and potentially fatal agranulocytosis, and so patients taking clozapine must have regular blood tests to check for this. In an OSCE, you may be shown blood results for a patient taking clozapine and be asked to interpret them.

Vignette

Mr C is a 35-year-old man with schizophrenia who has been taking clozapine for 1 year. He had his full blood count taken this morning for monitoring, and you receive the following results later in the day.

	Result	Reference range
Hb	14.0	13.0–18.0 g/dl
MCV	85.0	76–96 fl
Platelets	200	$15–400 \times 10^9$/L
WCC	3.8	$4–11 \times 10^9$/L
Neutrophils	1.2	$2.0–7.5 \times 10^9$/L
Lymphocytes	2.3	$1.5–4.0 \times 10^9$/L
Eosinophils	0.05	$0.04–0.4 \times 10^9$/L
Monocytes	0.2	$0.2–0.8 \times 10^9$/L
Basophils	0.0	$0.0–0.1 \times 10^9$/L

Questions

1. What would you do with these results?

   Clozapine should be stopped if the WCC falls below 3.0×10^9/L or the neutrophil count falls below 1.5×10^9/L. This patient's neutrophil count is 1.2×10^9/L, and so his clozapine should be stopped. A discussion should take place with the patient regarding alternative antipsychotic treatment.

2. How often should patients on clozapine have their bloods checked?

   Full blood count should be monitored weekly for the first 18 weeks after treatment initiation. It should then be monitored fortnightly, and if blood counts are stable after 1 year, it can be monitored every 4 weeks.

Mental Health Act 2007

Although it is not necessary to know the entirety of the Mental Health Act 2007, there are certain sections that you will be expected to know and that you could be asked about in relation to any clinical scenario. It is important to understand that the Mental Health Act is only applicable to patients with a mental disorder and it is only concerned with the assessment and treatment of the mental disorder itself. It does not cover the treatment of an unrelated physical disorder.

Section 2	Psychiatric admission, for assessment
	• Duration: 28 days
	• Treatment for the psychiatric illness can be given without consent under Section 2
	• Usually converted to Section 3 if longer admission is required
Section 3	Psychiatric admission, for treatment
	• Duration: 6 months
	• Treatment for the psychiatric illness can be given without consent for the first 3 months the patient has been under a section (including any time under a Section 2 before the Section 3) but, after that, consent from the patient or a second opinion appointment doctor (SOAD) is required
	• Can be renewed for another 6 months and then for 1 year at a time
Section 4	Emergency psychiatric admission when a second psychiatrist is not available, for assessment
	• Duration: 72 hours
	• Treatment for the psychiatric illness cannot be given without consent
Section 5 (2)	Emergency holding order (by doctor) for patients already in **any** hospital
	• Duration: 72 hours
	• Treatment for the psychiatric illness cannot be given without consent
Section 5 (4)	Emergency holding order (by psychiatric nurse or doctor) for patients already in hospital undergoing informal treatment for psychiatric disorder
	• Duration: 6 hours
	• Treatment for the psychiatric illness cannot be given without consent
	• During the 6 hours, a doctor must sign a Section 5(2) or the patient can self-discharge after the 6 hours
Section 57	Covers treatments requiring consent AND a second opinion
	• e.g. surgical implantation of hormones to reduce male sex drive
	• e.g. psychosurgery
Section 58	Covers treatments requiring consent OR a second opinion
	• e.g. ECT
Section 62	Covers urgent treatment
	• Overrides the requirements of Section 58 if urgent treatment is required, e.g. to save the patient's life or to prevent the patient from violent behaviour
Section 117	Duty of the local health authority and social services to provide aftercare to any patient that has been detained under Sections 3, 37, 47 and 48.
	• The patient does not have to accept the treatment (in contrast to a community treatment order)
Section 135	Removal of a person from his premises to a place of safety by the police
	• Duration: 72 hours
	• Treatment for the psychiatric illness cannot be given without consent
	• The patient must be discharged after assessment or detained under Section 2 or 3
Section 136	Removal of a person from a public place to a place of safety by the police
	• Duration: 72 hours
	• Treatment for the psychiatric illness cannot be given without consent
	• The patient must be discharged after assessment or detained under Section 2 or 3

Index